MY BODY AND OTHER CRUMBLING EMPIRES

MY BODY

AND

OTHER

CRUMBLING

EMPIRES

Lessons for Healing
in a World That Is Sick

LYNDSEY MEDFORD

BROADLEAF BOOKS

MINNEAPOLIS

To Mommy, Grandmother, Grandma, and all the women of my lineage, who've always deserved to heal and not to hurt.

CONTENTS

FOREWORD

I am fluent in multiple languages. In high school I studied Spanish and did my best to make fun of our *profesora* while retaining enough vocabulary to keep my dream of studying abroad—which, by the way, never happened. In college I switched to French, fueled by White saviorism and a vague dream to do community development work in West Africa. But these are not the languages I speak.

In early 2009, without signing up for a course or traveling across an ocean, I was plunged into the total immersion language program of chronic illness. In a matter of days, I started learning syllables I had never heard before. Burning. Throbbing. Stinging. Stabbing. I was twenty years old and a junior in college, and suddenly I could barely walk, hold a pen, open a book, or pray a prayer. The land of ease became a memory. The body I had implicitly used to make myself exceptional went on strike until I recognized her as more than a machine.

That year, I started learning the language of my body. I started listening to the phonics of my physicality. I started paying attention to parts of myself that Christians had taught me to fear, silence, cover up, and control.

Your body speaks in syllables of sensations. She (or he or they or ze) speaks through sighs, groans, tingles, and aches to tell you the truth about how safe you feel to show up in your life. Far too few of us have been given permission to learn the language of our limbs and longing. And, as Lyndsey Medford so stunningly shows us in this book, the powers of empire prefer it that way.

Today I noticed a stack of papers peeking out from the bottom of my bookshelves. They were notes from an American urban history course I took in the fall of 2009, just six months into my "language school" of liminality in my body. As I thumbed through the looseleaf papers, I realized not only that my handwriting has become *much* worse in the last nearly fifteen years, but that I was surveying the property lines society has set for power, privilege, and our physicality. I was locating myself within systems, society, and history in a way that would empower me to reposition both my body and others' bodies to no longer be commodified, crushed, and controlled. If we don't know our location, we cannot seek anyone's liberation.

Many, many years ago, a poor young woman on the brink of her whole future was surprised by a divine messenger, who invited her to bear in her body a Love who would change the world. Mary consented to become the mother of light, even though her consent would position her further outside of her society and religion's places of power. Her fear became a song.

The mother of God sang of the reversal of power. She reveled in the restructuring of society. She made the feeding of the hungry the chorus of her consent.

God entered the world through the womb of a woman who knew and rejoiced that the birth of love would become freedom for the oppressed.

My friend Lyndsey Medford has written us a song like Mary's. She has returned to the birthplace of Love—the human body. In consenting to a story she would never have written for herself, she has repositioned her own relationship with her body, her God, and her world.

I met Lyndsey through a writing mentorship I led a few years ago, where I witnessed a woman who not only has potent words to share but has the courage to live a life that matches them. I've watched Lyndsey live with integrity. I've seen her honor her body as more than a machine. I've noticed her humility to listen to those society has long silenced. In an industry where many writers hustle hard to be heard, I've watched this woman create for the sake of a joy and liberation that are unified with joy and liberation for her own body and all marginalized bodies.

The integrity I've seen Lyndsey cultivate is the integrity she invites you into in these pages. In the fierce landscape of loss and the crumbling empires of commodification and consumerism, Lyndsey has become so fluent in the language of wholeness she can translate our bodies' truths. She welcomes us home, not to a world where weakness stands knocking and orphaned at the door, but where our whole selves have room to stretch and rest. Learn her language and listen, for your body is speaking the words we all need to hear to be whole.

—K.J. Ramsey, licensed professional counselor
and author of *This Too Shall Last, The Lord Is
My Courage,* and *The Book of Common Courage*

INTRODUCTION

There is a whisper we keep hearing; it is saying we must build in us what we want to see built in the world.

—Sonya Renee Taylor, *The Body Is Not an Apology: The Power of Radical Self-Love*

Sixty percent of US adults live with a chronic illness.

Some of us take a pill and forget our illness altogether. Some of us are totally disabled. Some of us were on the couch today. Some of us should have been, but couldn't afford it.

Some of us have found amazing support from health professionals. Some of us navigate a confusing, unfair, and uncaring healthcare system. Some of us have little access to healthcare at all.

But all of us live with a before and an after. A chronic disease is a constant companion. Even if our condition is well-managed, some part of us knows that fragility and uncertainty have taken up permanent residence in our lives. We have all known what it is to be deeply grateful to a body, and to wish for a different body and, maybe, to do both on the same day.

We all experience not only our own lives but also the rest of the world differently than we did before. We wonder how much to reveal to our coworkers, families, or friends. We take health and healthcare personally. We have a different relationship with words like "need" and "dependency." We hear people declare confidently how to "be healthy," and we wonder what people like them think of people like us.

We are 60 percent, but too many of us feel alone.

Having a chronic illness—like any suffering in this culture, really—feels isolating and scary. Sick people end up feeling self-conscious. We're told we're unusual, or failures; it seems like a downer or an embarrassment or a weakness we should never show. We wonder if we're "complaining" too much when we're honest about our lives; we fear being stigmatized and stereotyped; we might accidentally make others uncomfortable if we joke about bodies and doctors.

But the truth is, we are 60 percent. More of us live with these realities than don't.

At the age of twenty-six, my childhood rare, chronic autoimmune disease—Behçet's syndrome—suddenly overtook my life again. I remembered that I am one of the 60 percent. At first, I thought the biggest long-term effect on my life might be adding more doctor's appointments to my agenda. Then I kept not getting better.

I've decided to spare you the suspense: "Healing" may be in the title of this book, but my illness is not gone. It's still chronic. I might even venture to say it's a part of who I am. I know how to manage pretty well, but that doesn't mean I'm healed. After five years of healing work, I'm okay with that.

Because even though I don't have certainty about how to navigate within so many limitations, I am certain my body and my life are good.

I believe we, the limited, matter, and we belong.

I believe we, the fragile, can show a culture of bravado how to live with finitude.

I believe we, the delicate, contribute something to the world just by being right here, on our couches. Again.

I believe we are canaries in the coal mine of a breaking earth, and our embodied existence, our boundaried lives, our networks of care offer prophetic presence to the world.

Over and over, my body, with its disease, has drawn me together with others. My illness is usually invisible, but since I started sharing about it with others instead of hiding, I've discovered I'm surrounded by people who also live with invisible physical or mental illness. For every person who makes it clear they do not want to engage, there's someone else who finds comfort and connection in sharing their own hidden experiences.

When we connect with each other, we can remind each other of the truth: We have all learned something about ourselves and the world from our bodies or our experiences. What we need matters, and who we are matters, and we deserve to be honored, cared for, and listened to, and to know we are never alone.

I am no longer a person who can chart a direct path to a goal and will my way to meet it. I am a dropout from every competition I once tried to win: the race to the top of the career ladder; the unending, unwinnable beauty contest; and even the secret dream of being known as a really, really good person—the best person, maybe. I don't have the energy to win any of those games; even when I thought I did, I didn't. I live week to week and day to day with such uncertainty about what my capacity will be that I don't have the luxury of making grand plans and strategizing my way to an ambitious deadline. My planner has great faith in me, but I can't follow its hand-lettered instructions to simply "make it happen."

This is not to say that I never again want to be successful, feel beautiful, or do good. It's just that the ways I was taught to define and achieve those things no longer make sense in the world as I know it. Ever since they stuck a planner in my hand on the first day of second grade, I'd learned to choose and chase external goals—all the skills of ordering my world so that my efforts would add up to the correct final sum (92 or higher, to be exact).

The thing is, I no longer order my own world. The thing is, I never did.

———

Your body contains two entire immune systems.

The first one is called the innate immune system, and it's your first line of defense. It's a network of cells that responds when you get a cut or encounter a familiar pathogen. These cells do things like clear away dead tissue and gobble foreign materials whole.

The second line of defense, the adaptive immune system, is more complex and subtle, and allows all the "learning" your body does to recognize and fight various (and even entirely novel!) pathogens. The most specialized of its cells, T-regs, are made in your bone marrow and travel through your thymus, a gland in your chest, to receive their marching orders. Then they reside in the lymph nodes in your neck, armpits, chest, belly, and groin until called upon by the innate immune system which sounds an alarm and calls them up against an enemy—or even against one of your own cells that's gone awry.

Among these cells, some subtypes can only be produced when certain bacteria are present in the gut. The bacteria signal cells in the gut lining, which signal the thymus to signal the newly arrived cells to "take on the T-reg identity."

In the midst of all this complex chemical signaling, sex hormones also play an important role. For example, pregnant women are advised not to eat sushi because their immune systems are suppressed by certain estrogens their bodies are producing.

If you're already confused by everything I've said about the immune system, don't worry—your doctor might be too. It's so enormously complex that science is still working to describe, let alone understand it all. What we call the "immune system" isn't much like the cardiovascular or digestive systems, with specific organs playing clear roles in the human body. Instead, it's an incredibly complex network of cells that, by their very nature, can travel throughout the body and must interact appropriately with any number of "self" and "non-self" objects and characters.

It's often likened to an army, but it could just as easily be considered a vast and intricate dance conducted by the music of biochemistry. At one moment in the symphony, the dance might dabble with some gut bacteria, or in another dramatic climax, it could involve the elimination of a cancerous "self" cell—long before it can cause any harm. Every day, the dance passes through and sweeps into itself the lymphatic, endocrine, reproductive, vascular, and digestive systems. The dance not only *keeps* us alive by keeping us from getting sick; in many ways the dance *is*, at least in part, our life.

To take a step back, though, what science has learned about the immune system mirrors a truth we all intuitively understand: It's a tricky balance to defend ourselves from getting hurt while also remaining open to what can help and nourish. Let down your defenses, and you'll end up serving a tea party to an enemy; over-police your boundaries, and you'll expend valuable energy on hostilities toward friends. There are a number of flaws in the popular idea of "boosting" your immune system, but the main one is that bigger isn't always better. An overzealous immune system might interpret peanuts or grass pollen as deadly enemies; it's like the Hulk smashing up a building over a piece of burnt toast.

You don't want a hulking immune system. You want a Tony Stark, Ironman-style immune system, capable of sorting through vast amounts of information to calibrate a precise response to your environment. And by and large—even if your body, like mine, gets it wrong a lot—a Tony Stark immune system is what you have. Your body can protect you from viruses, bacteria, parasites, and more, recover from entirely *new* pathogens, and heal itself while you go about your daily business. And it's the very complexity of the immune system, tied to its diffuse interrelatedness with your body's *other* systems, that makes it so effective.

Still, every Ironman suit has its limits, and even our miraculous bodies are evolved to survive in a different world from ours. Have you ever been in or heard about a college dormitory where everyone suddenly got sick at the worst possible time—finals season? That's because stress hormones signal our immune systems to dampen down, which is a good move if you need your energy to escape a literal attacker or find food. It's less strategic when you sleep, eat, and study in close proximity to hundreds of other people and really, really need to take an exam free from the influence of cough syrup.

In this case, the complexity of the immune system (specifically, the feedback loop between your body's stress response and its release of T-cells and antibodies) works against you. Highly complex systems are wondrous to behold, because their design allows them to do so many things, absorb so many shocks, sustain themselves in so many situations.

But if the self-regulating, self-healing functions of any system are taken for granted, it may continue to work—until suddenly it doesn't. The system may shut down, or its own mechanisms may even begin to backfire. Depleted resources, eroded emergency stops, or feedback loops gone awry can cause extreme unintended effects. When I took Naproxen every day as a kid to prevent inflammation, it eroded the lining of my stomach. Then my doctors told me to take Prilosec to counteract the resulting ulcers. But decades later, my stomach still doesn't regulate its own acid levels well—thus causing potential problems through the entire digestive system, thanks to the Prilosec that was supposed to *solve* a problem caused by a drug that was supposed to solve a problem.

We witness other systems gone haywire in similar fashion when we talk about the earth's greenhouse effects, misinformation going viral online, or pandemic "supply chain issues." The twenty-first century is exhilarating and overwhelming because the systems within which we live have become more complex than ever. Since the pandemic began, we're acutely aware that our lives balance at the intersections of forces well beyond our control—natural ones like disease; human-made ones like the vast scientific infrastructure that produces vaccines; even cultural systems like ideas about science, freedom, and democracy. These systems' vastness and their intricacy embody so many of life's paradoxes: they're simple but also complicated, resilient but also fragile, subject to laws and patterns but also unpredictable, wondrous but also terrifying.

Much of what we talk about when we talk about "social justice" depends upon a working understanding of systems like these and a willingness to recognize that context matters. Individual acts of service or charity could mitigate some of our world's problems, but justice means recognizing when the problems are being caused by our own collective choices about how to interact with and organize the world. Individuals who overcome obstacles can be inspiring, but justice means striving for a world where we don't put unnecessary obstacles in each other's way. Individual effort is laudable, but justice is when an imbalance of power or privilege doesn't cost anyone ten times the effort to achieve something.

Structural imbalances—ones we must work together on a society-wide level to address—are not only unjust, they're increasingly difficult to ignore. Many systems we've taken for granted are headed toward collapse. Many people who've long been oppressed are now in full-blown crisis.

We know that each of us plays a tiny, tiny part of our own in all these systems, but they seem too big, too old, too powerful, too far removed, or too hard to understand to participate meaningfully in them. Sometimes, the more we learn, the smaller we feel.

This is a fantastic place to be. After centuries of creating and interfering with these ever-more-complex systems, by rights humanity should be humbled and awed. Instead, people in power act with hubris that would be laughable if it wasn't so destructive. Feeling helpless or giving away our power isn't good—but smallness also isn't inherently bad. Those of us with a little perspective on our place in this world might have more clarity than some who've grown too comfortable wielding the levers of power.

When I first started trying to understand my chronic autoimmune illness, I had the same unending feeling of overwhelm. What is an "immune system"? At the question, anthropomorphic blobs resurrected from some childhood viewing of *The Magic School Bus* or *Osmosis Jones* helpfully presented themselves in my mind. Many of the layperson's explanations I read in books or articles offered similar non-answers in the form of metaphor. By the time I could pass the quiz about whether interleukins acted more like soldiers or assassins, I'd simply expended all my chronic illness "spoons" memorizing information that still had no reference point and no use to me.

For a long time, I waited passively for someone smarter and surer to rescue me. But there was never going to be an easy answer. Instead, I needed *both* to cultivate even greater respect for the power of my immune system *and* to claim agency and take responsibility for my part in tending to it.

My understanding of the immune system became a *working* understanding when I stopped trying to comprehend its every detail and instead began to appreciate its complex interrelatedness with the rest of my body. It's not actually a regimented, self-contained system like an army or a super-powered smart suit. It's a system like a global weather pattern, a school of fish, or even a church community: incredibly, beautifully complex, interdependent with other systems, wise and even mysterious—and powerful enough that when things go wrong, they can go horribly, horribly wrong.

As I came to know my immune system less as something I could ever hope to *control*, and more as something I participate in, I began interacting with that system with more care, respect, and intention. I had to begin that long (and ongoing) process well before I felt ready, knew where all the resources would come from, or even had any clue that it would "work."

Meanwhile I learned all I could about race and racism, economics and climate change, community, church, and social change, spent two years in the South Carolina Poor People's Campaign, and met other activists around my city and around the country. Under the mentorship of others committed to actively pursuing justice over the long haul, I found myself bringing the same habits of respect and intention to my interactions with social, economic, political, and environmental systems that I did to my own immune system. I could never control or even fully understand any of them, but I could fundamentally alter how I played my part in them, and help shift them from places of destruction to places of healing.

When it comes to my own body, I've experienced every inching step toward healing as pure gift. One of the most fundamental tasks in "claiming agency and taking responsibility" has been to ask for and accept help from all quarters. From the authors of books to my husband, Nate, who's always so ready to help me rest; from my doctors to the many friends who've offered encouragement, advice, and support; from yoga teachers to disability Twitter—at every juncture I owe my healing and my life to someone else. From my body to ancient writings to the voice of Holy Spirit, I owe it also to wisdom from well beyond my own mind.

I believe this is how we will *all* move forward: together. As Howard Thurman and Martin Luther King Jr. described in the phrase "beloved community"; as Black queer feminists have continually expanded upon; as so many global Indigenous traditions teach; and as Jesus in the Gospels and Holy Spirit in the Acts of the Apostles show us, the "power of love" is not a metaphorical or purely spiritual reality. Our interconnectedness is a force of nature all its own.

When we're deeply reintegrated within relationships that were broken—with our bodies and ourselves, with God, with our neighbors, with the earth—we are repairing and restoring webs of life that are the most fundamental, precious, and powerful systems in this universe. We are building solid, just, and kind foundations upon which to organize, march, and strike; deep wells from which to draw throughout the grueling work of change; flexible, resilient networks for the unpredictable future. We are touching what it means to be human and alive: sometimes small and often in pain, but also occasionally creative and kind, and always slowly remembering the outrageous truth that we belong, as Mary Oliver says, in the family of things.

———

But why do we so easily forget that belonging? Disconnection runs through patterns of commodification and objectification that reach into every area of our life and society. For centuries, our collective life has been structured around colonization, a system that never ended but only morphed into toxic, extractive capitalism.

Those systems, and the cultures that endorse them, constrain our ability to even imagine a good life or a good world beyond the metrics of production or consumption. We don't remember how to locate ourselves as more than isolated atoms bouncing from achievement to achievement. We wish for communities of deep trust, but we settle for relationships of niceness. We've lost our knowledge that the earth is not just a collection of raw materials but a place of unending interrelationship—a wondrous, creative, and kind home.

By the time I got sick, my theological education had taught me a lot about that history, and about what was wrong with the world, but I didn't know a way forward. I wanted to be a part of the solution, but the problems were too big. Why was it so hard to find a place in the food system where land, animals, workers, and eaters were all honored and nourished? Why did it take so long to find a doctor who respected the wisdom of my body like I did? How did it seem normal to spend my early twenties running on adrenaline until stress used me up and left me on the side of the road like a spent firework?

Voices from some childhood Sunday school classroom told me to either blame myself and myself alone—after all, I did forget my reusable grocery bags last week—or blame "sin" or "the fall" as if they were gravity-like forces we'd all have to just accept. That childhood theology didn't speak a language of systems, interrelationship, or community outside the cordon of the church building. It had adapted to the atomized individual and the insular comfort of the suburbs.

But sin is much more than my personal failings or a mysterious force. In *The Very Good Gospel*, Lisa Sharon Harper draws on her research on Genesis 1 and 2 to show that "sin is anything that breaks the relationships that God called *tov me'od* [very good, perfectly in right relationship] in the beginning. Sin is (and causes) separation."

This definition applies to some of my Sunday school sins, like stealing someone else's animal cracker, but it also encompasses much more. Sin is present anywhere we live in patterns of distorted relationship, separation, and isolation. The Law of Moses even provides for priests to give an atonement offering for unintentional, communal sin. Sin results in distortion and separation—which requires attention and repair—whether it's caused by the intentional choice of a single individual or the accidental neglect of an entire nation.

Communal sin shows up wherever human rights are neglected, bodily supremacies are invented, violence is done, or indifference slowly destroys. Communal sin keeps us trapped in cycles: unjust and inhumane cultures and systems teach us unjust and inhumane habits and relationships, so that we come to perpetuate those systems without even realizing it.

To break the cycle of sin, we must be aware and engaged on large-scale and personal levels—and often communal or institutional levels in between. We must become practiced at locating ourselves within systems and power structures, even and especially those that aren't designed to be seen.

The Bible does this when it insists that repairing injustice requires centering on the needs of widows, orphans, and immigrants—groups of people who were vulnerable within their society. God measures the righteousness of God's people by the well-being of those with the least power and status. But too often, God's people neglected those on the margins of traditional power structures, believing some in the community could flourish apart from others. The same happens today when our society fails our poor neighbors, our Black, Indigenous, and People of Color neighbors, our queer neighbors, our elderly neighbors, our caretaking neighbors, our women neighbors, our essential-worker neighbors, our immigrant neighbors, our unhoused neighbors, our neurodiverse neighbors, or our chronically ill and disabled neighbors.

Learning more about communal sin and systemic injustice should empower us to take responsibility for creating change. But often it makes us feel more overwhelmed and powerless than ever. We are shaped by so many forces outside our control; our actions can have so many unintended consequences; the problems are so massive and so long-standing, we wonder if it's even worth hoping things could shift.

But sin is not the beginning, middle, and end of the story. Sin is only a distortion of the story that is truest about our world: that life overflows in abundance when we are in right relationship with God, with one another, with ourselves, and with the world. These intricately woven, interconnected networks of relationship are indeed overwhelming when they've been twisted by greed, pride, and injustice. But they also, despite those odds, overwhelm us with beauty, grandeur, resilience, generativity—with the often-surprising sense that to be small amid a forest is not such a bad thing; that to be embedded in a community, however complex and confusing, is to be deeply at home in the universe.

The ancient biblical writers illustrated what modern sciences are finally coming to understand: that each being in this world is shaped, constrained, nourished, and inflected by every other. In God's garden, this is a beautiful and miraculous thing! But when greed, hubris, power-hunger, and hatred interfere, the grand and glittering web is twisted and broken.

Distortion and separation hurt so much because they're not the truth of who we are. The truth is that we are constituted by one another, materially made up of the world around us, and spiritually nourished by connection. God created the world's natural and human systems as dynamic, *interdependent* interrelationships. The flourishing of one creature can't be separated from that of any other. In our deepest being, we don't just long for health, peace, and happiness within ourselves; we long to be in loving and just community with our families, our neighbors, and our planet. Goodness resides within each of us, but it also exists *between* us.

Lisa Sharon Harper describes "God's dream for the world," this state of justice and peace among "a web of relationships that overflowed with forceful goodness," and names it as *shalom*, the Hebrew word for peace. I refer to it using one translation of *shalom:* Wholeness. In doing so, I deeply do not wish to imply that if we are not physically "whole" or feel emotionally or spiritually "broken" we cannot live out God's dream for us. Instead, I want to point to an opposite reality. Despite what individualism, consumerism, and capitalism tell us, we are interdependent down to our very being, and we only experience true Wholeness when we experience relationships that are radically *for* the flourishing of others. By reminding us of this truth and drawing us into interrelationship, our weaknesses, losses, and lack can actually lead us to greater Wholeness than that of the person who *seems* to have it all together, but does so alone.

Wholeness is like "integrity." A shorthand definition for "integrity" might be "truthtelling" or "honor," but the word itself paints a more vivid picture of a well-integrated person whose life is accountable to their values and supported by a deep internal consistency. For me, as I've come to include my relationships and communities in my definition of my "self," integrity also extends to being well-integrated in my family, friendships, and communities—even when it would seem less messy and more neatly bounded to keep a safer distance.

The truth is, we are not only connected; we are made of each other. We are made of dirt. We are made of rivers and bacteria and we breathe in gasses breathed out by grass. We get our vitamin D from the sun and our ability to be "good people" from those around us who love us and help us feel safe.

We are trained to "make something of ourselves" by straining and striving for independence. But the truth is, our selves are given to us, not made by us. We can't tend to ourselves without actively caring for one another. We can only make sense of ourselves by attending to the places we are woven within the fabric of relationship. Like our selves, like our immune systems, our Wholeness finds us in an ever-changing, dynamic dance of life.

———

When I began to recognize how I'd burned out my own body, I couldn't help but notice how many of these lost connections and skewed relationships within myself mirrored illnesses and imbalances in the wider world. Often the changes I needed to make for my own health also led me to healthier, humbler, more holistic attention to broader systems within which my body and life are enmeshed. At each halting step of incremental healing, I found that this baffling, invisible immune system was calling me more fully into my own humanity but also into a relationship of greater Wholeness, justice, and peace with the world: with my physical body and with the healthcare, economic, social, and food systems, in particular.

This book tells the story of how I am finding my own way to my own kind of healing, but it's not a book of step-by-step instructions for how to heal our bodies or fix injustice. Instead, I want to ask us to reconsider how we relate to our bodies and selves, communities and cultures, systems and ecosystems, from our internal dialogues to our neighborhoods to the global industries in which we work. If we're going to unlearn burnout, we have to let go of the myth of an empire-wide solution to be handed down by experts or politicians. We must reclaim our own power to uncover even the tiniest piece of the puzzle or pick up a small corner of the load. We must relearn to see and honor the wisdom, needs, and resources already present within every person, group, or place.

This is the kind of change that constantly asks us to question, to listen, to notice where our world is begging to heal itself—rather than to be fixed by our clever solutions. This transformation will draw us into faithful action and sacred relationship within ourselves, our homes, and our communities first, until we slowly realize that together we've grown templates for offering the same things to the world on a much larger scale. adrienne maree brown reminds us that this model of transformation and growth already lives within us:

> When we speak of systemic change, we need to be fractal. Fractals—a way to speak of the patterns we see—move from the micro to macro level. The same spirals on sea shells can be found in the shape of galaxies. We must create patterns that cycle upwards. We are microsystems. . . . Our friendships and relationships are systems. Our communities are systems. Let us practice upwards.

This is a book about practicing upwards. But first, it is a story about burrowing downwards—deep into my cells and my soul.

PART I

1

MY BODY AND OTHER CRUMBLING EMPIRES

I asked Jesus into my heart at age four. And five, and six, and seven—after all, there didn't seem to be any harm in making sure the process took. Even though the grown-up at the front of the room assured us all that the prayer had saved us, I never felt any different. Eventually I took this to mean that it had worked when I was four, and I just didn't remember what my sinful former life had been like.

But, though my soul was safe from hell, questions continued to abound, like How, exactly, did Jesus get into my heart? If Jesus was in my heart, why didn't he talk to me more? Was Jesus cramped in there? This last one occupied more of my time than you might think—I asked Jesus into my heart with roughly the same regularity that I watched *Aladdin*. I wondered if I should set Jesus free, like Genie

from the lamp, instead of cursing him with "PHENOME-
NAL COSMIC POWER . . . itty-bitty living space."

Long after I'd accepted the explanation that my "heart"
was actually some vague metaphysical idea, and "Jesus living there" mostly just meant that Jesus and I were friends,
I still wondered why grown-ups thought this heart thing
was an adequate metaphor. Sometimes I put my hand over
my heart to feel it *thump-thump-thumping*, wishing Jesus was
actually that easy to feel; as badly as Jesus had wanted to
move into my heart, I couldn't tell that he'd done much with
the place.

It was 1999; I was probably on my fifth or sixth salvation. I was in Dr. Tim's pediatric office, a familiar enough
place. But today I wasn't here for a fever or a cough; it was
the skin ulcers. They were yucky, I was deeply ashamed of
them, but they were also painful and they scared me, so I
told my mother and she'd brought me here.

Usually Dr. Tim told us what was wrong and prescribed
big pills. Today, instead, he kept asking us questions, then
frowning at his papers. I waited patiently for the adults
to decide what to do, confident they would make things
better—that was, after all, their job. Suddenly Dr. Tim
excused himself, and my mother and I were looking at each
other, in the little room, for the hundredth time. I'd already
studied all the contents of the cabinets and drawers. I sat
on my hands, wishing for markers, to draw on that smooth
white paper covering my table-seat.

A long time later, Dr. Tim burst back into the room with
a paper full of notes. He didn't know how to pronounce
Behçet's syndrome, but he knew what to do next. I tried
to listen to a flurry of information and the long list of next
steps he offered my mother, but none of it made sense
to me. Why would my ulcers be a clue that I might have

arthritis? I heard the words "blood lab" and started gearing up for a panic attack. They referred me to an eye surgeon. They had no suggestions for making the ulcers go away—what we came for.

The diagnosis—plucked from the depths of Dr. Tim's memories of scrawled med-school notes—would be a gift. Listen to stories of autoimmunity and you'll learn I am approximately the first person ever to wander into a general practitioner's office and walk out with a correct diagnosis and course of treatment. Most folks file through the offices of specialists for months, years, before they get an answer. Even more importantly, the subsequent battery of tests revealed inflammation of the iris, a condition that can go unnoticed until it causes at least partial, irreversible blindness. My sight and my mother's diagnosis-seeking sanity, we owe to Dr. Tim.

But it would take me a few years to accept that a diagnosis is not actually a cure; that there are things adults can name but not change. A "syndrome" is merely a name for a pattern of symptoms—an acknowledgment that you are not crazy—a sketchy roadmap of your future based on the medical histories of your far-flung, rare-disease-lottery-winning peers. A syndrome is a bewildering array of bricks flung through your window, and no one is under any obligation to help you make sense of them. Once you're diagnosed with a chronic autoimmune syndrome, most doctors revert from offering you healthcare to providing disease management. These diseases are confusing, often cyclical, and under-studied. Many physicians have admitted in surveys by the American Autoimmune Related Diseases Association: "I'd rather not see these people."

So at age nine or ten, I took on the task of learning to live with my illness. In due course I did receive a tube of gritty paste to dab on the ulcers while I bit my lip to contain whimpers of pain. The paste would help the skin heal, but it didn't prevent the sores, and it had to be cleaned out and reapplied in the same tense lip-biting ritual several times a day. I missed school regularly.

And I learned how to escape. I read with actual ferocity, willing myself to partition pain while I escaped to Narnia, or the 1800s, or an interplanetary future. My body was attacking me, I'd learned; but luckily I knew how to retreat.

As I retreated into books, it logically followed that in a house with several Bibles for each person, I'd also retreat into religion. Church is all about things we can't see or describe very well. It's all about ideas, which turned out to suit me pretty well, and it's about things I didn't yet understand, like "having Jesus in your heart," but which the adults seemed confident about. My family went to church two or three times a week; church rewarded you for knowing the right answers, like school. I was good at school. Maybe someday I'd understand Jesus and Behçet's syndrome too.

Wandering into my teenage years, I cobbled together my own interpretation of the heart dilemma. Having Jesus in your heart meant knowing as many Bible verses as possible, remembering that God is always watching you even in your thoughts, and being very nice to everyone. It was about interpreting a complicated world through the proper categories, and knowing "The Right Thing to Do" as a result. The evangelicalism of the '90s and aughts confirmed my personal suspicions: bodies are unimpressive and unreliable, but the mind can be taught to pray; a body will let you down, but the mind belongs to God.

By the time I was eighteen, my illness was in remission, a fading memory. But the suspicion and general distaste it helped engender for my body remained. Then I took up Muay Thai boxing to impress a boy, and I went to theology class.

My theology professor at the Christian college I attended said one day that "asking Jesus into your heart" is not a major concern of the Bible. It was, of course, disturbing to hear that my childhood teachers were spreading such misinformation, but it was also a bit of a relief. At least now that we were adults we could admit we were using confusing terms to talk about vague ideas: in this case, salvation by "the indwelling of the Holy Spirit."

Except, as Professor Skip went on to point out, "Holy Spirit" can be as simple or as complicated a term as we want to make it. While people have argued for millennia over the workings of the Trinity, Spirit has always most fundamentally meant—in Hebrew, Greek, and English—"breath."

This same professor would also be the first to suggest we might mean something about God when we talk about "creation" and "incarnation," that the story of God might have to do with more than just saving souls. Take Hebrew law, for example—what to do, how to arrange things, whom to care for—not that much in there about how to get saved.

The psalms and the proverbs, too, don't talk about people as souls apart from their bodies. It's all one thing, the human: the body needs its breath and the breath its body, and that's all there is to it. When you consider things this way, it's impressive how we've complicated these lumps of clay walking around. And it seems like getting your soul saved might not mean divorcing your body, after all.

The more I thought about it, the more plausible it seemed that God might even be up to more than just saving souls. In Skip's class, we imagined that God didn't create the universe just so people could screw it up and God could fix it. We considered the idea that maybe God likes the universe;

maybe God likes the universe so much that God would've been born into it even if people hadn't screwed it up. Maybe "God so loves the world" means that God loves the world, not that God loves "my heart."

Sometimes I'd go from theology class to the dingy boxing basement and let all those abstract ideas and overwrought words melt away. There was only the next punch, the sore shoulders, the dance. There was only the sound of my breath.

When I resurfaced to the wider world and my own over-thinking mind, I realized I'd just experienced the truth of those ideas: God might really be here, matter might actually mean something, and my body might be part of me—more than that, it might actually be me.

It's almost enough to make you mad. All this time trying to describe what it's like to know a God who is as big as the sky, as free as the wind, and as near as your chest, I'd only known how to say heart (but not your real heart)—when I could have just asked my breath.

Suddenly my childhood religion was cracked wide open, and we were no longer spirit-people, hurtling toward the day when we could finally leave our sad embarrassing bodies to join the spirit-realm. Suddenly we were here, here and now, for good reason—because it was a good place to be. Redemption had a new life for my classmates and me: it meant the renewal of all the world, the trees outside and our childhood homes and the dirty oceans and the crumbling neighborhoods across the railroad tracks, and this was a more tremendous thing than the earthquake-raptures we once imagined, because this thing tasted like hope.

Over the next years of unanswerable questions, my mind would unlearn, many times, how to pray. God and I picked up and left off at odd intervals while I failed to understand. But in all my most lucid moments, though I couldn't pray in words, I sat, inhaled, and exhaled. I would breathe until I could remember I was not alone. Where the sermons no longer reached me, Spirit and my own body could still my heart. I think that to be friends with Jesus is to know this: there's a little bit of Spirit in every drop of air, and every breath is a saving grace.

In those years, as I discovered that I needed and no longer feared my body, I also discovered the world. I began to wear new eyes. I didn't skim over things, uninterested in the non-spiritual, or suspicious of anything that drew me with too carnal a force. Now I went out of my way to stand under the ginkgo tree on Centenary Street in the days its petal-leaves began to fall, because I knew that only a sacred being could worship in such perfectly brilliant yellow.

I delighted in all sorts of material things I'd once feared to love too much. In the depths of a historic Boston winter, I realized again how thoroughly exercise could stave off my seasonal depression—and return my abstract theology student self down to earth. I studied the environment and understood for the first time that the natural world I'd always loved is not a place I visit but the planet I depend upon and live within. I backpacked through the mountains of North Carolina with a new sense of wonder, gratitude, and sacredness. And as I worked in a food pantry, then studied theology and justice in graduate school, I saw how subversive and how spiritual it could be to honor our neighbors' physical bodies and provide for physical needs.

Only a few years passed between my first thrills of love for my body and the first time my knee buckled under me, unleashing a cascade of symptoms that diverted my attention from bodily excellence to daily survival. But in those years, my body taught me much that I came to know about God and about how to be myself. I once aspired to approach creation with some detachment, in a rational but rather sterile fashion; now, I saw God plunging hands into earth to craft a world out of clay and play and a dash of Spirit too. I did meet God, all the time, in my own breath. I exercised, delighted in sex, felt everything just for its own sake, exultant and young.

So the sudden and debilitating return of my disease was all the more like a lightning bolt through my life.

————

For most of my life I've been told that my body is defective. Worse than defective, really—at times it seemed my body was perverse, belligerent, and almost obscenely . . . wrong. Once, I watched a betta fish dash its own bruised body against its tank, over and over, to spite the enemy in the mirror. Like that fish—doctor after doctor explained to me—my body attacks itself.

Behçet's syndrome, like any number of autoimmune diseases, mostly serves as a shorthand for a baffling collection of symptoms, little-known and not at all understood. In my case, its vascular inflammation causes mouth ulcers, genital ulcers, arthritis, and massive fatigue. It could also cause blindness, digestive issues, aneurysms, and neurological symptoms, and it could spontaneously go back into remission again at any time.

I know many people must search and document and fight and pay dearly for diagnoses of weird diseases, and they feel immense relief when they find one. But for me, it's always felt a little like knowing my precise location in Alice's Wonderland—a bit of an illusory sense of belonging or control. It seems the only relevant information I have remains:

1. I've fallen through a hole.
2. We're all mad here.

The number of people diagnosed with an autoimmune disease is rising by the day. I admit I have mixed feelings about our growth in numbers. Having a weird-ass disease is incredibly lonely; it helps that awareness of chronic illness has risen in the twenty years since I was diagnosed. I'm forced to explain myself less; for example, most people no longer take it upon themselves to judge whether fatigue is a real symptom of a real medical condition. And, while I don't wish for any of my friends to be stricken with nonsensical ailments, it is nice to know people who've similarly experienced the struggles of chronic illness.

Yet the rise in numbers also often leads me to despair. Everyone knows someone with an autoimmune disease—not even just "The Big Ones" like lupus or type 2 diabetes, but something weird, fascinating, and tragic. Those most eager to tell me this rarely understand that it's not an interesting personal quirk to have multiple friends with these ailments; it's increasingly a statistical likelihood. Researchers are beginning to use the word "epidemic" to describe the growing prevalence of autoimmune disease.

Still, that hasn't translated much into research or resources for us. There's no 5K for bizarre and barely treatable inflammatory syndromes (it wouldn't fit on the T-shirt). No decades-long, multi-billion-dollar quest has been launched to understand the cause of rising autoimmunity, as society has done with heart disease or cancer. Doctors, patients, family, and friends are still likely to chalk these diseases up entirely to a lightning strike of genetics—unconsciously settling around us an aura of terrifying unluck and inherent unhealth.

From the moment I knew at age twenty-six that Behçet's was back, I expected I'd get back to normal soon. It was 2016; that year I'd applied and been rejected from PhD programs, gotten married, moved in with my husband, moved from Massachusetts to South Carolina, and adopted a puppy. We were supposed to be young, adventurous, starting our new life together. "Medical science has advanced in the last ten years!" I said to my husband, Nate. "Surely they'll have a drug that'll fix this right up." But months wore on and nothing really helped.

This was inconvenient. Not only because I struggled to ride my bike or have sex or, some days, get off the couch, but also because I was knee-deep in all this "bodies are awesome" stuff. It was increasingly difficult to square this disease with my belief that God's creation is very good; that our bodies are ourselves; that the body itself, like the Bible, is a place of revelation. A body that attacks itself, betta fish–style, didn't seem to fit into that theology.

At the very least, my betta-body should have cooperated with all the drug treatments thrown my way. Instead, my body threw them up, laughed while nothing changed, conjured fascinating new side effects, or raged that much harder. I felt more and more like we were in a tug-of-war where either way, I lost. This body, this mass of dysfunction and pain, couldn't possibly be *me* like I'd said. I was supposed to be enjoying my twenties with my new husband and new puppy in our new city. *I* had no interest in this sad circus of symptoms.

At least, I thought I didn't.

But several months and several drugs into this ordeal, I began to ask: Was there any possibility my body knew some reason for it all?

I remembered dealing with depression in college. After a bad breakup in my senior year, in 2012, I'd been plunged into a cloud of despair. After several months, with the help of friends and family, I emerged hopeful and grateful—and also certain this monster would be back someday. I'd had to ask myself: When it returned for me, was I going to fear the monster and resist it, deny its existence until it knocked me flat on my back, or was there a way to befriend it?

I saw that in the depths of depression, I'd ignored and hidden my deep exhaustion, soul-level sadness, and crushing loneliness—and that I might not survive by coping the same way again. My body and mind had been asking me to slow down, to get help, and to connect with loved ones.

I'd responded by working harder and isolating myself more.

In retrospect, my depression symptoms pointed not only to immediate needs but also to deeper issues in my life that required my attention. It took long months, first of suffering from depression and then of recovering from it, to come to these realizations. I held my relationships and myself to impossible standards, to the point that a bad breakup with the boxing boy made me feel like an existential failure—like I was stranded. I was desperate to prove my worth by hustling hard, and I coped with my grief and self-blame by trying to appear all the more hardworking and self-sufficient. In my hyperfocus on achievement I was terrible at practicing vulnerability in relationships, leaving me trapped in suffocating shame I thought I had to hide from even my closest friends.

Depression was the most unequivocally awful and unendurable thing I'd experienced in my twenty-one years—but it eventually pushed me into the unfamiliar practices of self-kindness and vulnerability. Ultimately, in the process of tending to my symptoms and asking why they showed up in the first place, I came to appreciate that my body and mind had been offering me deep wisdom, if only I'd been humble enough to accept it. I needed to slow down, process my emotions, and connect with others after the breakup. When I refused to consciously do so, my body had done the best it knew how: to take the rest it needed and release its emotions through sleep and tears, sleep and tears, sleep and tears.

The next time depression appeared, I was determined to give my body and heart the attention they demand by seeking the help of a counselor but also by offering kindness and ample space to my needs for rest, support, time, and patience. I'd ask my body what it needed from day to day, in hopes of giving my soul the space to discern what was draining my life away and bringing me to this place of collapse.

It wasn't until I rejected the betta-fish narrative, imagining peace with myself in place of war, that I realized I could ask my physical illness the same thing.

The immune system is an incredibly elaborate, and still poorly understood, network of defense against disease. It has two main components: the innate immune system, or first line of defense from foreign objects and organisms, and the adaptive immune system, which recognizes and destroys invaders and aberrant body cells with far more precision. Each component involves entire phalanxes of cell types dedicated to functions as diverse as forming mucous membranes to keep foreign objects out, responding to and cleaning up after a paper cut, learning to fight a new virus by creating more white blood cells specifically targeted to it, and recognizing and silently destroying a tiny cluster of cancerous cells lurking within the body long before it can cause noticeable damage.

We've all experienced pain and suffering at the hands of our own immune systems. When you get sick with a fever and headache, or suffer from redness and swelling due to a sunburn, those symptoms aren't caused by the pathogen or the sun damage themselves. They're side effects of the immune system's massive mobilization to prevent further damage and begin the process of healing. And they're not just the regrettable collateral effects of that process; they serve an invaluable evolutionary function. Fever alerts us that something is wrong and that our bodies need us to slow down. Resources are slim while the body is focused on warding off catastrophe, and we need to muster them judiciously, not head off to the climbing gym. Inflammatory pain from an injury, likewise, signals that we need to take it easy while the repair process is underway.

Autoimmune disease is generally characterized by inflammation that's gotten out of control with no discernible cause. Conventional medicine responds by moving to suppress the immune system. "Nothing is wrong," we try to tell the body. "Simmer down." But as I began to accept my autoimmune body—moving toward it with more curiosity than condemnation—I wondered whether I should take my immune system at its word that it was trying to protect me. What if something *was* wrong?

As I researched autoimmune disease, I learned that many conditions are genetically programmed but don't show up until a life circumstance like a nasty virus or traumatic event causes the gene to "switch on" and express itself. Normally the immune system is self-regulating, so the body can efficiently clean up and return to normal after the war-zone experience of inflammation. But when autoimmune disease appears, the immune system has been sent into overdrive, or stayed for too long in active battle mode instead of its usual stand-down patrol; the gene is activated; and suddenly overdrive turns into hyperdrive. The brakes on the system no longer work, and its painful, inflammatory services to the body become chronic symptoms interfering with everyday life.

I hadn't experienced an obvious triggering event, either as a kid or as an adult. But when I started asking how to support my body and respect my immune system, rather than immediately labeling it a problem, research turned up several factors that could be triggering immune reactions.

My doctor had never even suggested that there might be factors besides genetics and bad luck conspiring to keep me sick, but by paying close attention, I began to see patterns. When I asked my body if she was trying to share something with me—the same way I'd learned to greet depression—she answered. My symptoms improved when I avoided certain foods. I had more high-energy days overall when I took care to slow down on low-energy ones. I came to notice that my joints held stress within them as pain and inflammation and learned how to process stress better. I also made hard decisions to help avoid it; I practiced yoga and gave up, at least for a while, on working full time.

As a kid I'd been told that, as the Bible says repeatedly, "creation reveals the glory of God." My body belonged to creation; over time I'd come not only to believe but to repeatedly experience that bodies are places of divine revelation.

When I felt tangled up in a personal problem or a writing conundrum, I could go on a long walk in rambling or wordless prayer and almost always return with some small thing settled into place or something unimportant having fallen by the wayside. When I searched frantically for direction in life, my body would kindly request that I return to the present moment and drink a glass of water—and often, in the process, to return to enough equilibrium to notice the one tiny "next right thing" that might lead me forward. When another person made me angry, defensive, or sad, I could ask questions of those sensations and thank my body for its information about what was important to me.

Likewise, when I dared to believe that God had not left my sick body but that her signals continued to be gifts to me, it turned out that my body had not betrayed me. When I offered my body compassion and curiosity and gave her what she needed, she was ready and waiting to heal. I had betrayed my body by treating *her* as an *it*—a tool to be used for work, a sculpture to satisfy someone else's gaze, a machine to be fueled with the cheapest possible food, an inconvenient nuisance of a reproductive system, but rarely as a precious ally and friend, deserving of exquisite nurture and care.

I'd followed the cultural script laid out for me by working sixty-hour weeks during grad school to prove how responsible I was; overexercising to prove how desirable I was; applying to PhD programs and getting married and moving across the country and getting a puppy all in one year without a breath or a thought or a therapist because I was twenty-six and I thought that was what you did. I'd been drawing, perhaps for years, upon resources I didn't really have. My autoimmune disease may have been a genetic fluke, but it was also a classic case of burnout.

In response, my immune system did what it was designed to do: protect me, in the only way it knew how. It directed its fury at food particles I couldn't properly digest, signaled that my stress levels were destroying me, and desperately struggled to offset artificial chemicals that continually kept my hormones out of balance. Its hyperactive responses in turn clamored for attention toward my body's needs. But

I was young and busy. I didn't think of my body as having needs. I responded to my immune system's protective alarms with anger and contempt; I impatiently took myself in to a professional exactly like a car needing repair instead of a miraculous organism in need of loving care.

Now I had to practice meeting my body like a late-repentant lover, like a car person approaches an Aston Martin, like a guitarist reverently opens the case on a Taylor. Anything that requires so much maintenance and care must be special. Just as Nate and I were learning in those first years of marriage to speak up about our needs instead of suffering silently, my body created enough friction to force me to take notice and make things better.

Instead of trying to fix a broken body, I was now repairing my *relationship* with systems I'd forced into overdrive. Alongside the help of science and medicine, I began to trust my body herself, as a complex, interconnected organism, to seek her own balance and healing. And as relationships righted themselves within my physical body, relationships among my mind, body, and soul had to change too.

2

WHY WE NEED TO HEAL

Even if I really thought God was speaking to me through the signals of my body, I can't exactly say I wanted to listen at first.

I didn't want to know how distorted my relationship with myself was. I didn't want to unlearn a quarter-century of beliefs about being a "good person" or a healthy one. I didn't want to investigate my gut bacteria or delve into my belief that my productivity mattered more than my joy.

A whole chorus of voices in my head constantly chimed, *try harder, do more.* Only months in a state of collapse could cause me to even realize I was burned out, let alone question those voices of self-exploitation. Until then, it didn't occur to me that I didn't know who I was—or even who God was—without them. Only my body, who literally could not try harder or do more, could gently pry those lies from my hands and teach me (internally kicking and screaming) how to just be.

I probably thought I already knew how to "be kind to myself," but it took years to truly learn how to care for myself with the attention and compassion I needed. For many, many months I'd find myself straining to perform an obligation, complete a chore, or even do an exercise routine that I hadn't really decided, for any reason, to do. It was an expectation I'd taken on automatically because I thought I "should" be able to. I ended up with a hard-won mantra: It doesn't matter what you should be able to do. What matters is reality—what you are able to do.

I had to stop looking for external markers to define my responsibilities and measure my successes. I had to continually name that my healing process required time and effort; I started saying chronic illness was one of my part-time jobs in answer to the dreaded "what do you do" question.

After years of reorienting my habits and my definitions of success, and of talking to other women dealing with physical and mental burnout, I've even had to name that healing itself is a countercultural practice. We're all taught to view our bodies as machines and our sicknesses not as natural processes, but as mechanical failures. No one is applauded for staying home from work when they're sick; even children are rewarded for having perfect attendance at school. It doesn't matter that you might get more done in three days working, after two days resting and making a full recovery, than you would in five days of sitting miserably at your desk. It's the admission, itself, of weakness that's viewed as failure. We're taught from our early years on that we should fear self-indulgence more than self-destruction.

I'd never put my well-being over work before, and having the ability do so at all drew on so much economic privilege (among other kinds) that I struggled to imagine I "deserved" it. Jesus said, "From everyone to whom much has been given, much will be required" (Luke 12:48 NRSV). I was supposed to be starting a career in nonprofit work, not cooking myself finicky meals and then collapsing from the effort. It took a long while to accept that, while much *had* been given to me, much had also been taken from me. It took even longer to entertain the thought that *I* might be more than those ever-expanding expectations and my ability to meet them.

It was hard to trust that I could devote all my time and energy to my own healing, not least because I come from long lines of frontier-chasing White people who prize hard work and self-sufficiency above all. I was not raised to view "healing" as its own activity that could occupy any time or energy—let alone years of my life. I was raised to be gritty, determined, and masterful at masking pain. I was expected to work so hard that my privilege could hide behind the veneer of my progress and perseverance.

The practice of turning to my body with compassion was therefore unfamiliar, unwieldy, and uncomfortable. I was unceremoniously forced to recognize that my autoimmune disease didn't make me a diva but a human being with needs. At its deepest core, my disease was asking me to reckon with my physicality and my finitude. I had loved my body when she was strong; now I faced the true test of loving her when she was weak. I had theoretically known I lived within concrete limits; now I ran up against them nearly every day.

Alongside the slow and painful process of physical healing, I had to heal my relationship with myself. Could I respect myself when I couldn't live up to the mythical American dream of infinite progress? Could I love myself as I was, at this particular place, in this particular body, in this particular pain—and not as I'd once dreamed of becoming?

Nate, my family, and my friends loved me, not hypothetical future me. They offered me space and time to rest without any expectation that I'd "make up for it" later. They cared about how I was feeling, not just about what I could do. At times I was the last person in the world to accept that I was terribly ill. I could only do so because the love of my people—most especially Nate—showed me how.

It felt like a loss to grieve my previous belief in my own infinite possibility, but it also opened up *new* possibilities to accept my limitations, embrace my smallness, and recognize my interdependence with others. When my resources shrank so drastically, I had to consciously choose between priorities instead of pretending I could "prioritize" them all. Living squarely in the midst of what was instead of what "should" be felt like freedom—especially in those areas where I hadn't even realized I was operating out of a "should" mentality. Once I realized I couldn't live up to most of the societal expectations for how bright, privileged twenty-six-year-old women live their lives, I could finally consider how *I* wanted and needed to live my life.

I had never offered myself the acceptance and generosity to believe that my needs, let alone my desires, mattered very much. It felt daring to believe that I could trust my own body, offer care to my own heart, and receive exactly what I needed—even when my needs seemed extraordinary. Until, after an immense amount of practice, it didn't feel that way anymore; it felt normal and necessary. The less I was able to chase what I thought others expected of me, the more I could simply pay attention to what was emerging from my own truest being. What did my body need that day? What information were my emotions and desires generously offering me?

I'd begun spending more time in yoga practice, bringing my fullest presence to postures that drew energy, balance, and strength from solid foundations, attentive alignment, and ever-flowing breath. My cardiovascular fitness and muscular strength were waning, but I could still stand on a mat and breathe; and my body showed me there was more to her than just the ability to exercise more and more vigorously.

Sinking into a deep stretch, my hips remembered how flexibility can only slowly, steadily grow through release. Tottering in a balance pose, my core muscles engaged to bring stillness from energy, from center. Turning the world upside down, my legs found movement flowing from solid, connected foundations. Shedding suspicion and embracing trust in myself began to feel like that in the rest of my life: flowing from a deeply centered way of being.

I'd thought letting go of external ideals and rules for myself would make me feel like a sailboat adrift on the open ocean. Instead, it felt like knowing where home is for the first time. When I discovered that my body knew what I needed to eat to feel well, all the made-up diets I'd spent my life following suddenly appeared ludicrous. When you only have energy to do a few things in a week, there's a galvanizing force to the kind of clarity that brings.

In my experiments with living this way, I also discovered I brought a less scattered, more centered, more present self to the people and places that mattered most. I could no longer entertain the seemingly humble, but actually self-important, belief that I was responsible for everything and everyone; instead, I had to leave everything and everyone up to God. In the space left by that recognition, I could see in bright outlines and hear in deeply resonating calls those few places I was responsible for being deeply, fully present.

I quit fretting and strategizing to "balance" all the things I thought I was *supposed* to care about, and simply did the things I cared about. We spend so much time telling each other that we're more than our appearances, our finances, or our work, but every single time we push beyond our limits to meet invented standards for those things, we teach ourselves and everyone around us the opposite. For the first time in my life I actually sat down with myself and my family, drowned out the manic noise of "everyone else" (whoever that is), and discerned what mattered to me about my body, my finances, my work.

Most importantly, as I slowly unclenched my fists from invented ideas about what I "should" be able to do, I also began to release their darker shadow side: questions and accusations about what I deserved to have. It didn't matter anymore what I deserved. It mattered what I *needed*, regardless of whether or not I was able to "earn" it.

In accepting my need for care, I slowly let go of my shame around how my privilege enabled me to rest, eat nutritious food, and receive compassionate healthcare. Instead, I started asking with renewed urgency why *everyone* in the richest country in the world couldn't meet these simple needs. The books I read about treating my disease with "lifestyle interventions" always stopped right there: with *my* individual lifestyle. They assumed I'd be able to find organic food, spend time in nature, and pay for regular doctor visits and lab tests. Even though they were written for individuals, I was always surprised they didn't at least acknowledge that all these things took so much effort and resources, in part because our systems made it so.

It helped me cope when I remembered that I was learning entire new ways to interact with those systems—and even, in tiny ways, to help change them. I didn't see my disease as my fault for "unhealthy" habits, or improvement as my reward for the changes I'd made. I'm a theologian, trained to look at everything within its broader context. I couldn't help noticing how my illness stemmed from patterns of relating with the world *outside* me, not just inside my cells.

Reorienting to new habits led me to ask how my skewed relationship with myself mirrored other distorted relationships in the world. All the things that had triggered my disease were just regular aspects of a life I considered "normal." But did that mean there was a problem with me? Or was the problem with normal?

I had used and abused my body rather than encountering her as a sacred space. After all, this is what we're taught: to control our bodies from early ages, to play through pain, to conform to outside measures of beauty and health. In our society, we are what we achieve; to need care, to slow the pace at all, is already to have failed. We often don't tend to ourselves or even ask if we're running in the right direction at all until we literally cannot keep going.

I even worry that, as we grow more willing to talk about burnout, we are coming to think of it as a normal part of every life or career, rather than a sign that something is fundamentally wrong with the way we operate. We struggle to imagine a different way of living and working because we've learned to see ourselves, and everything else around us, as engines of production and consumption, not as sacred beings in our own right.

———

Jesus was born into a nation under foreign military occupation. When he was a newborn, his family fled from an infanticidal puppet king of the Roman Empire. As an adult he lived, traveled, and preached within Roman society's matrix of strict social hierarchy. His message of liberation—love that could transcend this hierarchy by proclaiming the worthiness of all—eventually got him executed as an enemy of the state. His resurrection was God's victory over the forces of the empire—not victory through swords and wars, but erupting subversively from the most unlikely place: the lowest place, literally under the ground.

Rome occupied Palestine in order to extract its resources and accrue wealth, power, and security for the faraway Roman elites. But Romans didn't all see themselves as violent, destructive thieves of others' land and livelihoods. They believed they brought superior culture, religious and philosophical truth, and economic opportunity to the backward, provincial, perhaps even barely-human (they thought) peoples they conquered over the centuries. They claimed that their military dominance had ushered in a *Pax Romana*, benefiting the entire empire, because the superpower had ended wars by winning them all. This wasn't true; uprisings and all-out wars continued in various places. But the *idea* of the Pax Romana cast Roman supremacy as a benevolent force, and its enormous military as a protective (rather than a destructive) one.

To this empire, the death by torture of one Jewish man—even an innocent one—was at best an unfortunate administrative oversight, but more likely a necessary evil. An empire, by virtue of its sheer size, must be efficient, and to be overly concerned with "justice" would interfere. In light of its ultimate source of power—its violence—it must be brutal, and to be anything less could undermine its authority.

In history class we're told that the modern world has done away with invading empires and their supremacies. But as a US citizen and follower of Jesus, I am learning to tell the truth, in defiance of the lie of a *Pax Americana*. My country is built on stolen territory; I live on unceded Kusso and Kiawah land. Even after displacing and nearly erasing so many Native nations, the United States continued to expand through armed conflicts with even more sovereign countries, including the Mexican-American War, the invasion of the Kingdom of Hawaii, and the occupation of US territories.

This empire continues to enforce invented hierarchies of race, class, gender, ability, and others in order to funnel power, wealth, and security from the bottom to the top. It treats non-White cultures and people as disposable, poor and minority communities as occupied territory, and its own living land as an inert resource to be exploited for greed or burned through decades of carelessness.

My country is quick to enforce uniformity and call that "wholeness" or "peace." But in doing so, it actually shatters a peace that would include everyone—that would foster Wholeness for all. When children go hungry, prisons are better-funded than schools, refugees are turned away, and wildfires rip through overdeveloped and under-cared-for lands, we are not at peace. The vast majority of us are subject to a slow war of attrition stealing everything from our sense of safety to our powers of attention, from our labor to our lives.

Since colonists arrived in the Western Hemisphere to take away gold, since factories and corporations arose to alchemize human labor into profit, modernity has been defined by patterns of ever more efficiently using this world and each other. We've severed ties with our soil, our sense of place, our neighbors—and in the case of the powerful abusing the oppressed, with our own humanity. We have substituted superficial definitions of prosperity for the ability to recognize the sacred in each other.

In every place we lose our interconnection with the world, we both participate in and are harmed by sin. Failure to live in right relationship with God, self, creation, family, community, and the world are embedded in so many of our cultural habits and attitudes, systems of power and resource distribution, and public rituals and conversations. We believe power and wealth must be hoarded, not shared. We struggle to imagine prosperity that's not defined by overconsumption; leadership without domination; belonging that doesn't depend on someone else's exclusion.

It's no wonder sin can feel like an overwhelming force in the world; it is one. In all the places we hurt, we're longing for the re-creation and restoration of ecosystems of goodness and peace.

I certainly felt this sense of helplessness in my first years of being sick. Before, I'd been intimately acquainted with the insanity of the US food system but also so overwhelmed by it that I put off finding local and sustainable food sources in Charleston. I wondered often why we in the United States talked about healthcare only in terms of who pays for it, rather than ever bothering to define the words "health" and "care"—but without any expertise, I felt at a loss to define them even for myself. I raged against extractive capitalism, but I never imagined my labor, my time, and my life as things being extracted from me (by me) on behalf of that relentless engine, "The Economy."

I'd come to analyze things through a systemic lens, but under that lens it seemed like I represented only the smallest, and therefore least significant, unit in the system. I could recite the history of colonialism and detail how the most powerful country in the world had been built on greed, exploitation, and violence, but that massive systemic lens only seemed to underscore how little power *I* have in the world as it is. In this way, too, I'd left behind my childhood belief that the world would be better if we could just change enough people's hearts. Now, I'd rather change laws. Next to the power of legislation, my own private behavior seemed inconsequential. But that was before all those interlocking, exploitative systems came home to roost in my body.

———

I used to believe I'd escaped the worst consequences of the American insistence on commodifying everything, from sacred land to Black bodies and lives to water and time. That system of using everything up and throwing it away was designed to benefit me, an upper-middle-class White person. I never noticed how it was insidiously teaching me to use myself up and throw me away. Now, some days my knees and hips ache and I remember that my disabled body has been thrown into the vortex of all those systems' hidden costs, alongside poor people's bodies, disabled and elderly bodies, bodies of People of Color. But all those types of bodies can be, and are, also autoimmune bodies. And unlike my body, not all of them have access to the material resources needed to heal. I live with far fewer barriers to claiming my human right to health than most people in my country.

In these years of experiencing my body's dis-ease, I've ever-so-slowly learned to appreciate her ability to detect when something is wrong and insist that I pay attention. I no longer have the option of ignoring and exploiting myself for very long, pretending to delay the consequences

indefinitely. These days, when I feel her twinges and tired-
ness, I not only recognize that I need tending, I also feel her
calling me back into integrity with myself and right relationship with the wider world.

Likewise, all of the interlocking systems in which we participate are offering us clues that our extractive, exploitative
habits can't be sustained much longer. My body is only one
of those systems, but as I am still learning, it's a wise and
prophetic one. Glennon Doyle says some people with mental illness are like canaries in coal mines: "In a profoundly
sick society filled with racism, misogyny and all of these ills,
we breathe in all of these toxins (and) we get sicker." Autoimmune bodies are canaries too—sensitive to both literal
toxins and figurative cultural and systemic ones.

The good news is, the very complexity that makes those
systems so difficult to fix once they're thrown out of balance
also makes them highly resilient in the long term. My body
is not "cured" or returned to its previous state, but a hard-
won new normal has emerged through my doctor's care and
my reconsideration of my life choices, big and small. The
same is possible for our food systems, our healthcare systems, and more.

Jesus says our greatest power to resist empire and foster Wholeness doesn't lie in our ability to wield empire's
weapons—violence, economic exploitation, fear, and hatred—
for ourselves. It's not even in democratically wresting control
of the government that we are to place our hope.

We can be called to join the prophetic cry, "no justice,
no peace," because this is simply a description of our present reality, but the bitterness of injustice doesn't excuse us
from pursuing wholeness and peace. "The kingdom of God
is within you," Jesus says (Luke 17:21 NKJV). You have the
power to erupt through empire right where you are.

———

Just like there's no single magic pill for my body, no person, organization, or politician has the answer for making food or healthcare just and sustainable. Our systems' problems call for solutions as diverse and widely deployed as their causes. And that can be a good thing. We're so used to imagining power as a top-down proposition—as something some people have, and others don't—that we've been convinced to forget the power of small-scale but widespread transformation.

What I don't mean is small-scale but widespread *actions*. This is not the part where I try to convince you that our world's pressing issues call us, deeply and urgently, to a little recycling here and a trip to the farmers' market there. In fact, we have too often defaulted to well-intentioned but ineffective (or harmful) actions, tacking on more "virtuous" tasks to our to-do lists, because we don't remember how to *be*—or to become.

This becoming, if it is radical enough, will touch every aspect of our lives. It may ask us to reconsider our dreams, our worldviews, our worship. And at the same time— because it is so deep, taking place at a cellular level—it may at times look on the outside as if nothing is happening at all. That may very well be the case; for so many of us, an essential step in unlearning empire's colonizer culture is to practice surrender.

My own choice to seek out local, organic food won't change an outdated, unjust system; in fact, I could consume this food as a niche-market status symbol and likely do more harm than good. But when this practice is about belonging to a local food ecosystem, it can ask me more questions and call me to further action: to learn about the agricultural and labor practices of farmers and support sustainable farms, to advocate politically for community-led solutions to food apartheid, to begin a relationship with the land by cultivating the soil around me, or to share my table with my neighbors more often.

This way of relating to the world doesn't discount the importance of federal legislation, technological innovation, or good corporate governance; it just doesn't put all its hope in those tools alone. It dares to believe that what we need is not a few superhuman leaders, but millions of leaders whose very humanity is their strength. It trusts that when we align our small habits and big life choices with our own values and our own communities' flourishing, we will *also* find ourselves in the very specific place in the world we are called to occupy: one where our deeply intentional, interrelated actions can reverberate with the greatest impact.

The story of colonization, objectification, and exploitation can feel so long and broken that the ending seems like a foregone conclusion: we are destroying the planet, one another, and ourselves faster than we can even document our losses. No economic class is exempt from burnout. No place on earth will escape it. Too often our "solutions" seem to be little more than the invention of new industries to profit from the destruction.

But humanity isn't inherently destined for perversity and evil, any more than my body is. We're created good and indwelt by a longing for Wholeness. We can offer kind attention to the places crying out to be tended. We can wield creativity and love to reimagine our businesses, our farms, our cities, our countries. We have new technological, sociological, even psychological tools for growing kinder relationships and kinder systems, not just for making war and growing already-bloated economies.

Healing is embedded within our DNA and within the DNA of all of earth. What if, instead of resisting, numbing, or bypassing the signs of distress, we leaned in close? What if we gave our pain its overdue respect, and our innate, God-given wisdom its forgotten honor? What if we dared to believe that our communities, in the most unlikely, over-looked places, have already been given everything we need?

We could right our upended relationships from the cellular level, out.

We could become people who embody repair.

PART II

3

AMERICAN HEALTHCARE AND OTHER OXYMORONS

The day I hopped off a barstool and my knee buckled under me, I had no time to consider that my life might have just changed forever. I was hosting dinner for some new friends, and I had to walk the puppy first. Being new to town was exhausting.

The knee kept growing, reddening, and becoming more painful, but I kept having things to do. Since there was no reason for this to happen, it logically followed in my mind that I could will it to un-happen. It was almost two weeks— and my knee had nearly doubled in size—before I noticed an ulcer in my mouth. I suddenly and certainly knew what this was: Behçet's was back.

I couldn't ask any of my brand-new, twenty-something friends if they liked their *rheumatologists*; I'd be the youngest one in the waiting room by forty years. I picked one off the insurance list whose office was close to my house. She was curious and attentive. She confirmed my diagnosis and pre-scribed steroids to combat the worst of the flare.

After several weeks, the prednisone was helping, but ste-roids are hard on the body. We had to find something else. I slept, walked the puppy when my knee and my fatigue allowed, and adventured through the pill-of-the-month club, enjoying long philosophical debates with myself over which symptoms of the disease were better or worse than the side effects of the meds. Months went by this way. Work. Sleep. Wait for the next doctor's appointment. Eat.

After ten months, no drug I'd tried had helped me function at better than about 60 percent capacity. At the rheumatol-ogist's office I ventured a question about the autoimmune-allergy connection (allergies are a type of autoimmunity). "My pollen allergies have reemerged since we moved from Massachusetts to South Carolina," I noted. "Maybe that has something to do with why this is happening now."

"Maybe," my doctor said kindly. "Or maybe it was just time."

She meant to be helpful. She could hear me searching for some semblance of agency within this tiresome, frightening story. No doubt she was familiar with the mental gymnastics and quixotic quests of patients unable to accept the realities of aging and disease. She wanted to spare me the endless disappointments (and expenses) of becoming an easy mark for explanation after explanation, cure after cure. But what I heard was, "Don't try to understand. Your engagement is not necessary here. This was always ordained for you, and I am ordained to manage it."

People can genuinely intend kindness and still perpetuate cruelty.

I went home and started googling. Up until then, I hadn't wanted to know anything. I'd been convinced this was a minor setback the doctor would quickly sort out—no need to make a big deal about it. But I realized I needed to settle in to living life with this thing, so I set about conducting a background check on my recently arrived roommate.

It turns out it's a shady, slippery character. The scientific literature on Behçet's syndrome would take up slim space on a bookshelf. Some researchers have identified a gene or two and some specific types of white blood cells that malfunction in people with the disease. Beyond that, most of the articles I found reported on the efficacy of various immunosupressant drugs for treating Behçet's, sounding more like a naughty-and-nice list assembled on the fly than evidence of robust scientific inquiry into the actual workings of the body.

Opening a PDF of one literature review, I discovered I was reading an exact history of my own treatment. I was currently a little farther than halfway down the list of pharmaceuticals, presented in order from most effective and least side effects to more dire options. My doctor and I had dutifully tried each pill in turn, each pill in turn failing to help, or causing intolerable side effects, or both. I knew she was puzzled; she'd even made noises about sending me to the Mayo Clinic in Florida. But I hadn't realized my remaining treatment options were quite so bad.

I moved on from stalking my specific syndrome to trying to understand autoimmunity more generally. A quick local library search turned up one book that claimed that the singular answer to all my problems was definitely to eliminate caffeine and another that blamed iodine; another asserted that I definitely actually had Lyme disease; and one basically suggested that infecting ourselves with tropical parasites is the miracle cure the modern medical establishment has been hiding.

In this sea of overblown claims tinged with desperation, one book eventually stood out: *The Autoimmune Wellness Handbook: A DIY Guide to Living Well with Chronic Illness.* No promises of cures, just ideas about getting along better with this asshole roommate. No single piece of advice, but several small steps toward better supporting my body. No wholesale demonization of modern medicine—just the gentle observation that the suggested non-pharmaceutical "lifestyle interventions" generally have no side effects. The other books made false promises of control, but this was something humbler, and kind. This felt like the agency I'd been seeking.

Still, the book sat on the dresser, because I didn't have those words yet for why I might feel I could trust this approach. I still wondered about it like I wondered about all the other books: If these suggestions helped so much, why hadn't my doctor offered them? *The Autoimmune Wellness Handbook* suggested a drastic elimination diet that I just didn't feel ready to undertake. It also said I should go camping. I loved camping, but I wasn't going to become one of those people who claims fresh air is a better drug than prednisone.

I was still just trying to get this thing fixed.

———

Was it my sixth? My seventh visit to this doctor in all these months? *I wish they didn't make you sit in a high chair to draw your blood,* I thought, rummaging through my purse for something, anything, to fidget with. I gulped cold water from a paper cup and smiled at the other people in the room as if to calm them down. They were never as worried as I was; my body has a mild phobia of needles, my blood pressure sometimes dropping until jagged stars invade my vision and the world goes black. That day, my heart had already been racing, my head light for a while, since my doctor told me we'd exhausted our options in pill form and she was prescribing a weekly injection. *This is good, maybe this will be the one that helps,* my brain said. My body geared up to reject these future weekly wounds.

"Would you mind loosening this band? I've passed out before," I asked the phlebotomist, trying to sound nonchalant.

"It's a tourniquet. It's going to be tight," she snipped as she relieved the pressure choking my arm.

I was being treated like a complaining child, but I guessed I shouldn't be too surprised. Even when the doctor was kind and patient, she conveyed through her busyness, her degrees on the wall, her brusque responses when I ventured an idea, that I as a patient should sit down and shut up. When it came to managing my health, I was viewed more as a liability (prone to eat too many cookies or forget my meds) than as a partner; my familiarity with my own body, ability to read and research, and willingness to participate didn't count for much here.

The bloodwork went smoothly despite my insistence on retaining consciousness.

———

One of my favorite Bible characters goes unnamed. My Bible places her under a header: "A Dead Girl and a Sick Woman." How delightful. I wish we knew her name, but even without it, I recognize her. Pain has reduced me, too, to a bit player in stories that pass me by. Sometimes it feels like wherever I go, I am only "Sick Woman." I explain the long gap in my résumé and pray the interviewer for the job will still be able to see someone besides Sick Woman. I let the bread basket pass me by and suddenly I'm answering questions about all my symptoms and taking essential oil recommendations from a stranger. Maybe I'd hoped to be their friend, but I must play Sick Woman first. The doctors and insurance companies think they know Sick Woman, laugh about her when I'm not around, tell her to be patient, tell her to cheer up. Sick Woman tries to comply while Lyndsey waits to be seen.

The sick woman in the Gospel of Luke "had been subject to bleeding for twelve years, and she had spent all she had on doctors, but no one could heal her" (8:43). For a long time she fought the pain, seeking out one contemptuous man after another whose poking, instruments, tonics, and pronunciations were powerless except to slowly drain her purse as pain drained her life. Her houseguest's hostage, she tried to ransom herself but bought instead sneers, invasive examinations, more pain, and an unending cascade of blame.

Pain had taken her money and banished her from the temple; it had marked her for pity, disgust, fear, and now much of her life was a void. This is how it happens: Pain itself sidles into the void. Sick women are not believed, "but I believe you," croons pain. Sick women lose friends, "but I know you best," the constant companion says. So the memory of health fades into the distance and the promise of a future recedes even farther. The more that sick women are told we have imagined or caused our own suffering, the more we wonder if somehow we did want to suffer all along. We cannot remember whether it is mad to pull our pain tight around us or mad to hope for escape, so we do both.

The sick woman entered in the middle of someone else's story. Jesus had just arrived in her town when a "synagogue leader," a powerful and dignified figure among their people, ran up to beg Jesus for his daughter's life (Luke 8:41). A huge crowd had come to see the traveling preacher, but now he was on a mission for a powerful man, to save a little girl. His fame had grown; Luke says "the crowds almost crushed him" (v. 42).

A little girl was dying, but the sick woman had been bleeding for twelve years. Unlike many of the people Jesus healed, her illness—because it was related to menstruation—had rendered her ritually unclean every day of those twelve years. Women couldn't enter the temple's inner court, but menstruating women couldn't go into the gates of the Court of Women either, or even the outermost of the concentric circles, where non-Jews were allowed and which functioned as a market. Because they were unclean, they were utterly exiled from "tainting" any form of worship with any part of their community.

Jesus was often seen in the Gospels sparring with the leaders, priests, and scholars of his religion about ritual purity. It was central to their religion that everything and everyone belongs in a God-ordained place, and anything out of place is offensive to God. They weren't all gleefully ejecting people from the temple because they were cartoonish villains (although they may have come to enjoy the power of arbitrating who was in and who was out). They genuinely believed that God's design for Wholeness depended on maintaining strict order.

When Jesus argued with his fellow religious teachers about handwashing or minor Sabbath infractions, it wasn't just a fight about rule-keeping or even power (though it was also about those things). It was opening questions about the very nature of the universe. Was the civilized world forever teetering on the brink of chaos, requiring vigilant policing of boundaries to prevent sin, decay, and madness from seeping in? Or is it love, wholeness, and holiness that are even more catching? If we're willing to cross the boundaries that maintain our tenuous grip on order, could it be not evil but the kingdom of God that grows wild from a tiny mustard seed? Could it be rightness, safety, and belonging that reassert themselves, given the chance?

What I love most about the sick woman is that she didn't wait for these men to decide. She didn't care about handwashing *or* the nature of the universe. She cared about her own restoration to health and belonging, so she reached out for it. She touched only the hem of Jesus's cloak, and immediately she was healed. She was the one to violate the boundary, an unclean woman deliberately touching a holy man.

She felt it. She barely had time to make any sense of what had happened. She wondered for a moment if she was somehow dead, because she no longer felt pain. She was frozen in the jostling crowd, looking with awe at her own hand where it brushed him.

And then he stopped.

A little girl was dying, yet he halted. He was scanning the crowd and deputizing people to find her. He was insisting, against the insistence of everyone around him, that what she'd done mattered and that it should usher her into the center of this crowd.

Would he rebuke her, rescind her healing? Would he demand some sort of payment she had no way of making? Shouldn't he go to the synagogue leader's house?

She was not only overcome with gratitude and disbelief, but now also with fear. She stepped forward and collapsed in front of him as she told the whole thing—how his cloak had healed her.

"Daughter," Jesus said, causing her to finally raise her face to him, "*your faith* has healed you. Go in peace" (v. 48, emphasis mine).

A servant ran up to the synagogue leader. It was too late. *Don't bother the teacher anymore.* And here she was: bothering the teacher.

But he had just praised her. An hour ago, she was an outcast. Sick Woman. Now he had made her, in her courageous reliance on him, the hero of her own story. He'd declared that her audacity on her own behalf belonged.

He turned to the wealthy man and his servant. "Don't be afraid," he said to the terrified man. "Just believe, and she will be healed" (v. 49).

The penniless woman, at least, believed. So Jesus went on his way to take his life-giving touch to a dead girl.

———

I do believe in modern-day miraculous healings. And I used to pray for them as a kid, missing school or gritting my teeth against pain once again. I prayed to be normal. I prayed to be able. I prayed, too, for faith; I thought of the Sick Woman story, and tried harder to believe.

Back then, it was easy to look at the broadest strokes of stories like this one and take the idea that "Jesus wants everyone to be healed" to mean that Jesus only cares about the most whole, capable, put-together version of you. I would "reach out for my healing" in prayer because I wanted to be better for Jesus. And I would hide my pain, because it made it so much harder to "just believe."

But today, all the details of this story seem to point me in the opposite direction. I think this is a story about a healer on a mission to resist meeting those who are sick with the same fear and disgust as those who would call them "unclean." He was a healer for the penniless and hopeless woman—someone the forces of empire had discarded long ago—so accustomed to shrinking and hiding that she expected to encounter only a scrap of his cloak.

Jesus was not only willing or able to do this; he also interrupted his spectacular mission on behalf of privileged people to make sure her story was told. By his actions he declared that there is always time to witness healing and participate in restoration. By his words he praised the woman's resourcefulness. She violated a basic boundary of the religion he taught, and he stopped everything to look her in the eyes, call her his family, and tell everyone the good news. She was no longer Sick Woman. She was a faithful daughter—by the overreaching action she took while she was still cast out and unclean.

At my own most audacious, I wonder: Was Jesus really most impressed with her belief that some wild-eyed country preacher's clothing had magic powers?

Or was he also praising her faith—flying in the face of all the societal, religious, and medical narratives surrounding her—that she herself yet deserved to belong and to be well?

Living with autoimmune disease means living at the crucible of unlucky genetics and a hostile environment; outside the narrow set of circumstances where Western medicine is most successful; at the edge of a society that demands relentless positivity and has little patience for suffering that doesn't end.

Science pours money into clinical trials aimed at extending the lives of cancer patients by one or two years, but interest in non-fatal chronic illnesses—in improving the lives of people who may live with their disease for fifty or more years—is comparatively scant. Funding for environmental and public health, factors that could help prevent chronic disease, is even more scarce.

Life with chronic illness means sometimes feeling abandoned. But even when friends start assuming we're too sick and stop inviting us to things, even when our doctors run out of options (or interest), even when the drug is thousands of dollars a month, Jesus still stops and turns to place us at the center of a story about restoration.

———

After the demoralizing bloodwork incident, the doctor stopped me on the way out the door: "We will get to work on your prior authorization with the insurance," she said. The injections were so expensive she would have to make a special plea on my behalf.

Two weeks later, I got a phone call: The insurance company would pay for the drug, the pharmacy said. My copay would be 200 dollars a week, but the drug company might bring it down if I called them. I thanked the lady and hung up. I'd been thinking through these next steps, and it had been my best two weeks, physically, in the last nine months. At the suggestion of some friends, I'd been taking turmeric. It cost five cents a day.

I still take turmeric today, but it wasn't a magic fix any more than any other drug. What it did was *help* at minimal cost and with few side effects, and made me wonder what other simple supports might help my body restore itself after a flare.

I didn't want to try the next, expensive new immunosuppressant injection—at least not yet. (I would later learn that this class of drug works incredibly well for many people, but is also known to commonly work for months or years and then suddenly stop. No one knows why.) I'd been the subject of my doctor's failed experiments with medication for a long time now. I didn't *know* if there was anything else worthwhile out there; but if the best available treatment plan was trial and error, I wanted a stretch of time where the experiments were gentler.

My body had been met with suspicion, domination, and dismissal for long enough. As kind as my doctor was, she'd been trained in the same system of medical care that had trained me as a patient: the model where patients bring themselves in to be fixed like cars, where it seemed that all solutions were pharmaceutical solutions, where our own knowledge of our bodies and our stories is overwritten by a narrative about all that's wrong with us.

If you have an autoimmune disease, you don't hop on your insurer's website and get yourself an immune system doctor. Instead, you have a doctor for each symptom, and none of them speak to each other. At multiple points, I've had a rheumatologist, an ophthalmologist, a gynecologist, and a primary care physician, none of whom had ever heard of Behçet's disease. Our medical system trains physicians by body part, splitting patients into organs.

It also trains them to split us from our contexts. Doctors might take a family medical history, but they rarely ask about or evaluate so many other important factors: our physical environments, structural access or barriers to care, fresh food, or exercise, past traumas, cultural attitudes about bodies, health, and disease, or our bodies' experiences of acceptance or discrimination in the world. But every day when we live, work, and heal, whether we notice or not, we do it within all these matrices and systems that directly affect our bodies. A healthcare system that actually aimed for health and wholeness—for right relationships within the body and between bodies—would have to re-place us in our contexts, in our environments, and for most of us, re-locate us within our bodies, our selves.

I had to see if there was another way.

4

HEALING COMES FROM INSIDE OUT

Two years earlier, in 2015, Boston recorded four blizzards and twelve feet of snow. I was in my final semester earning a master's degree in theological studies, and I took one of the hardest classes of my life: a high-intensity interval training (HIIT) class for pass/fail credit. Between chapel and Constructive Theology, I sped up the hill on Commonwealth Avenue to the gleaming new fitness center full of gleaming undergrads and huffed my way through the boot-camp-style exercises. For the first time in my life I was unsure if I could handle a course and marked the final add/drop date on my calendar. As the date neared, each class session humiliated me and pounded every muscle into a rubbery lump of fiery lactic acid. Still, I decided to see it through for one reason: it made me warm.

Of course, by the end of the semester it had also made me strong. I'd never felt particularly capable as a body before, and I came to love the class with the wild eyes of a new religious convert. I was partly enthralled with the all-consuming experience of interval training: when you're entirely focused on pushing yourself through the next thirty seconds of lunge jumps, constructive theology sort of flies out the window. The class ended, but interval training remained part of my routine, up to three or four times a week.

Through graduation and a new job, through engagement and the wedding, through the move to a city I'd never seen, HIIT stayed with me. By January of 2017, I was trying to hang on to it through an autoimmune disorder too.

While my joints swelled and ulcers proliferated on my skin, I attempted to continue my high-intensity exercise habit with cartoonish zeal. The threadbare ability to complete a twenty-minute workout—though it zapped the entire day's energy—served as the major premise in my argument to myself that I was not all that sick and would be better within a few weeks. Every time I missed a workout, I could feel my strength ebbing. I didn't want to slide backward; I only moved forward! I'd earned this body by showing up to these punishing workouts *regardless* of how I felt.

One day, not up to squat jumps and burpees, I went for a jog instead. I counted mailboxes and waved at neighbors to help me pretend I couldn't feel my knee filling with a puffy ache at every step. "I'm home! My knee only hurts a little bit," I shouted at Nate as if shouting made it true. "Gooooood," he said—almost as if he knew he'd have to watch me pout, betrayed, the next day when it swelled and stiffened to become less like a joint and more like a knot in a tree.

Later I learned that I, not my knee, was the traitor; high-intensity training is all about pushing the body to its very limit. Demanding so much several times a week had become another stressor adding to the overload surging through my body, tipping my immune system over the edge in the months leading up to my illness.

If I'd known that it would in fact take years to heal, perhaps I would've given up interval training sooner—or perhaps, out of grief, I would've doubled down even further on my denial. That was, after all, what interval training helped me avoid (then, the next day, forced me to face): grief for the ease of my earlier years and for the body I'd barely yet come to know as strong.

I slowly accepted that my physical activity would be limited to walking. Meanwhile, the steroids calming my joint inflammation and slowing my skin ulcers also added twenty pounds to my small frame. As I began to look in the mirror less and less, and once burst into tears upon adding another pair of pants to the long-lost too-small pile, I eventually had to admit: my frustration and fear over quitting HIIT wasn't just about losing strength or a hobby.

I liked myself more when I was skinnier.

———

When your body is attacking itself, you're faced with a choice. Will you treat your own haywire systems as friend or enemy? I struggled to see my hyperactive immune system as more than a defect, the weakest link, a traitor. As a Christian theologian, though, I believed the human body, mind, and spirit can't be separated; to be human is to be all three, interconnected. Now it seemed my body itself was split down the middle, thwarting my will, sending my emotions into spirals. Was my theological viewpoint too neat to contend with the demands of reality?

It dawned on me that, from one perspective, the answer to the question of whether my body wanted to be my friend was immaterial. My feelings about my body were irrelevant. My religion requires me to love my friends and my enemies. I didn't have to settle the question of friend or foe; the answer, in any case, was to live and act with love.

To love my body. In all my years of yoga and inner emotional work, of interval training and backpacking breath prayer, had I ever once loved my body? Had I ever trusted it when it was inconvenient, checked in with its needs ahead of my mind's ambitions, or treated it as an end in itself—rather than as a means? Or had I merely pretended to love my body all along—the better to use her?

I realized I sometimes struggled to even find language for what it might mean to value myself, another person, or a place in and of itself, without reference to what it could do for someone or how it might be optimized in the future. My "body image" improved in my twenties because I'd come to appreciate how well my body could scale a climbing wall or bike a city. "Strong is the new pretty!" the Girl Power Internet chirped. This was certainly an improvement over my previous thigh hatred, but it wasn't self-love. I was still using my body, not inhabiting my flesh.

But now I was grieving activities I'd once enjoyed, perhaps even an entire life I'd once loved and a person I'd once been. Why should I also feel shame and sadness about my body's *appearance* when I had so much else to deal with?

I wasn't sure how to change how I felt, but I knew I could try to *act* with love toward my body—whether she turned out to be friend or enemy. In the process, I had to confront how often each day I judged my body based on its appearance, and how rarely I bothered to occupy it with tenderness and care. Now that my body wasn't strong anymore, I was less concerned with the new pretty. I didn't much care how others saw my body. I didn't need to improve my "body image." I just wanted to wake up and *feel* okay.

I was born with a genetic predisposition to autoimmunity; I wasn't born with an impulse to self-hatred that would be triggered at a certain weight. Where did that come from? Who decided my health struggles made me ugly? What did the volume of my fat cells have to do with the value of my body, of my self?

My academic brain readily answered: the cultural forces and systemic power structures of patriarchy warped my sense of self and conspired to keep me obsessed with smallness instead of growth.

Some more visceral part of me produced a river of images and feelings, one for every day of my life. They fluttered around me like my mother's sticky notes in her bathroom, meticulously recording each day's weight. Hours, maybe weeks lost willing the mirror to show a flat tummy; the stab of recognition and shame on the middle-school day I learned the word "muffin top"; workouts that promised to shred, shrink, destroy, blast, crush, flatten, or kill my body— the knowledge that I was the enemy.

I liked myself better when I was skinny. And now this was no longer a nuisance or something to "work on"; it was an absurdity. No—if it kept me from choosing my own body's side, it was a life-or-death emergency. Plenty of other things were attacking my body; I could no longer be one of them. My disease had drawn me into a fierce fondness for my body, and as I listened to her and defended her, anger blossomed within me.

Of course I'd known for a long time that my self-hatred served others' interests. But I treated this as merely an unfortunate circumstance, one I should be able to resist. I felt some vague shame at my inability to shed the obsession with thinness merely by not dieting, or by wishing to be confident. I didn't want to be an angry feminist, so I'd taken personal blame for a systemic issue.

Once weight gain forced me to see how easily I'd accepted my role as a victim, I bypassed "angry feminist" and become a raging one.

Around this time I also learned that the relationship between weight and health was far less straightforward than I'd always been taught. The disconnect I felt between my body's appearance and its actual health mirrors widespread issues in medical practice. Despite the fact that dozens of factors predict overall health and risk of serious illness and death better than body size, society still treats "fat" and "unhealthy" as synonyms. On the whole, the medical profession has ignored and denied mountains of evidence by perpetuating this stereotype—a bias that directly endangers the lives of thousands of fat people every year. Fat people are routinely turned away from medical care, misdiagnosed or under-treated, or outright shamed and denigrated by their doctors. Even though there is little to no empirical basis for assuming fat causes disease, and certainly none for the effectiveness of diets or of shaming people for their body size, anti-fat bias remains an acceptable stigma to hold against others, from cartoons to operating rooms.

Of course, the harms of anti-fat bias are even more dangerous for fat women, because bias against them compounds the stigmas and barriers to adequate medical care that all women face. As a sick woman, I was lucky to have the ulcers on my skin. If I'd merely gone to the doctor with joint pain, fatigue, and depression, I might not have received treatment at all. Ulcers were the one outward manifestation I could point to and definitively demonstrate that something was not right. The list of symptoms attributed, explicitly or implicitly, to the millennia-old catchall of "hysteria" (a Greek word for "wandering uterus") is long, but it doesn't include gaping sores.

I've always shied away from anger. It scared me a bit, and it seemed—as my old novels used to say—unbecoming. This time, my newfound body needs threw my old fixations into such sharp contrast, anger seemed the only sane response. Anger said: what I lost to patriarchy and diet culture for all these years *mattered.* My pounding heart and warm face reminded me: my body and my self are worth protecting from this nonsense. Rage gave the gifts of precious energy and unassailable clarity.

I had no more time to waste assessing my adherence to an impossible, imaginary, oppressive, arbitrary standard. No more ceding food and exercise decisions to some scowling godfather of not-good-enough. No more mental energy, self-confidence, or simple joy would be offered up on the altar of other insecure people's opinions.

I discovered that my anger didn't have to be all-consuming or blindly destructive, especially when I offered kindness to it instead of shoving it away. It was a force that wanted to flow through me, empowering me, then expressing itself, and subsiding for a while. Sometimes it seemed that for all the years I pretended not to be angry, I'd been overloading my reserves with one more helper-turned-toxin. But now, in giving space to its signals and cautiously trusting its lead, something inside me loosened a grip I didn't know I was holding. Before, I was seething uselessly, while suppression only added to my layers of felt helplessness. Now my anger and I were finding a necessary rhythm of power and peace.

Restoring my relationship with this aspect of my emotions helped me access empathy and connection with others. I sensed deep compassion at the core of my anger: for myself, for the women of my lineage, even for the misguided and disconnected people who actively perpetuated this culture of disdain for women and our bodies.

Anger also returned me, over and over, to *clarity* in the face of gaslighting and lies about the relationship between weight and health. There was grief in all of it, too, and joy at newfound freedom, but these didn't discount the importance of a healthy anger. Anger lends power and voice to the compassion at its core. All of these emotions have their place.

Later, when dietary treatment dropped my weight to its lowest in my adult life, I only grew more dedicated to my feminist rage. People told me I looked good, they made jokes about how tiny I was, and of course some part of me was gratified—but the larger part was grieving and angry. Friends could see my smaller waist; what they couldn't see was the year of pain and suffering or the fact that my diet consumed my life. I'd lost inches, yes, but I'd also lost the layers of muscle I moved to Charleston with. I didn't want to be congratulated for my diminishment.

———

When the doctor proclaimed that a weekly injection was our next best option, I decided—terrified of needles and unwilling to admit I was that sick—that I would give the drug merry-go-round a rest. By now I was utterly wrung out by the whole cycle of drug prescription, hope, side effects, trying to power through in hopes my body would learn to tolerate the drug, weighing disease symptoms against side effects in the world's least fun game of would-you-rather, and returning to the doctor in defeat. I just wanted a break from the treadmill as much as I actually had any faith in the *Autoimmune Wellness* hippie ladies' plans.

I called the rheumatologist. "I need to cancel my appointment," I said.

"Okay, when should we reschedule for?"

"I'll have to call back in a few weeks," I replied. "I . . . I'm gonna try managing this with diet and . . . stuff." The receptionist laughed through the phone at me.

So take what happened next with a grain of salt, because it's entirely possible I've gotten better just to prove the smug receptionist wrong.

The elimination diet was called the Autoimmune Protocol. By removing potential triggers and (literally) catering to the best of my 300 trillion bacteria, I hoped my body's inflammation could be calmed—so I removed from my diet all grains, dairy, legumes, eggs, nuts, seeds, sugars, alcohol, caffeine, soy, and nightshade vegetables.

Months earlier, this would have sounded absurd, but now I was coming to understand the absurdity of our medical system as it's generally practiced. Doctors are mostly trained to treat isolated body parts for common problems using pharmaceutical interventions. A systemic issue, a rare disease, one that doesn't respond to drug treatments? Three strikes—it seemed I was out of the actually-healing-people medicine game.

I'll try the weird diet, I told my own skeptical side, *and if it doesn't work, I'll march back in, accept my fate, and face my fear of needles.*

I almost quit the experiment after two weeks; nothing had changed except I already hated the sight of sweet potatoes and avocados. The regimen was kind of brutal—it turned every meal and every snack into this whole fraught production. I'd committed to the full twenty-eight days, though, in the spirit of scientific experimentation. Giving up was enticing, but I couldn't quite bear the thought of not knowing what could have been. It would be stupid to spend all this time and energy managing a disease if it turns out I just needed to not eat eggplants or something (I definitely hoped the culprit was eggplant).

It was the third week when I began to notice improvement. After eight weeks I felt better than I had in the year since all this started. And several weeks later, when I got stressed out by the whole thing and spent a weekend devouring ice cream and pizza, symptoms suddenly reappeared. I wasn't cured, and I didn't want to live this way forever—but I still felt my quality of life was better than at any time during my months of treatment with conventional pharmaceuticals.

Most importantly, I'd experienced that my body was willing and able to heal herself. Soon I was able to reintroduce some foods and discovered sensitivities to others—learning, in the process, how to pay closer attention to my body's signals. This didn't actually feel like dieting; it felt like lavish kindness and acceptance of my body and her apparently extravagant needs. This was what it felt like to be in a nurturing partnership with myself instead of a war. This was the kind of change that could take place with patience, care, and time.

I knew I still needed a doctor, but now I wanted to work with someone who looks at an unwell body holistically as something to be supported, rather than as a deviant to be contained, suppressed, patched.

I didn't know if a different approach to medicine would make me better. I knew I wanted to try visiting a medical professional trained in the art of listening.

My twentieth or thirtieth Google search unearthed a practitioner who took my insurance, and this is when I began to hope again.

My new doctor kept me on the immunosupressant drug that was half-working (and leaving me vulnerable to pathogens) while we searched for other symptom triggers. She was willing to follow my hunch that I may need allergy testing, and asked for a few extra tests besides the usual top eighty allergens. Dust, mold, cedar trees, and grass all activated my immune system, but we eliminated my worst fear—I wasn't allergic to the dog!

One of our earliest experiments was to stop the hormonal birth control I'd been taking for menstrual cramps since I left college. The debilitating cramps came back, but the debilitating autoimmune symptoms on the other thirty days of the month were cut in half almost immediately. Clearly, too much lab-created estrogen had kept my system out of whack until now. I started to feel almost normal again; I was riding my bike, starting a garden, and considering jobs.

While I was still far from "fixed"—still on a drug for transplant patients and struggling to follow a strict diet—the simplicity of this solution once again baffled me. Why had birth control pills been presented to me as the only option for coping with cramps or preventing pregnancy? Why didn't my rheumatologist care to know about this hormone-autoimmune connection? Why would we treat this massive change in body chemistry with such flippancy?

Birth control was convenient for my doctor, to collect my co-pay and get me out of his office. It was convenient for my husband (no planning, no condoms!). It was convenient for my employers. It seemed to be fine for other people, even for a younger me. But now I felt I wasn't given all the information I needed to make an informed choice for my body. I didn't love sitting on the couch trapped under a heating pad for two or three days a month, but I could plan around it.

I started preventing pregnancy by taking my temperature every morning to track ovulation. Over time, as I was reintroduced to my cycle without interference, I noticed there's a rhythm to my moods, my skin, my cravings, my need for activity, and my need for rest. I'm not a productivity (or exercise, or socialization) machine available at any moment to do any and every thing, but there are times when each of these comes naturally, when I can bring my best self to them, when I have a lot to give. They just depend on those other times my body asks for a few days of retreat.

I noticed so much about my body in those days. My body is not a machine; my body is not like all other bodies; my body is not like a man's body (or "deviant" from it); my body is not a hostile environment; my body is not easily divided into its constituent parts—and neither is my self: my body, heart, mind, and spirit.

But modern Western medicine has failed to notice many of these crucial facts about bodies. It gave me the steroids and immunosuppressants I needed to not be completely debilitated by my disease, but I had to search for someone who would help bring the many other available tools to the project of living at peace with my body in the long term.

My body also doesn't exist, move, or heal in a vacuum. Layers of privilege intermingle with layers of marginalization, overlaid onto my body whenever I encounter a healthcare system full of medical and wider cultural biases. In my woman's body, complaining of fatigue, I walk into doctors' offices knowing I risk being ignored. Or my doctors might have a baseline understanding of the human body drawn from research performed only on male bodies.

Recently, my long, irregular menstrual cycles and painful, heavy periods—which I faithfully mentioned at almost every medical visit, even with the same doctors—suddenly leapt to the forefront as an issue worthy of attention and care when I spoke the word "infertility." It felt like my desire to fulfill my womanly, procreative destiny had somehow earned me a pass beyond some veil where we finally admit that these symptoms are not "normal."

Even though women face immense amounts of medical discrimination, in my White woman's body I don't fear the rampant racism of the medical system—or of my medical providers, or the insurance company. As a cisgender body in a heterosexual marriage, I don't face judgment, fear, or misunderstanding about my experience of my body, my family, or my sex life. In my thin body, no one has ever suggested that my knee pain is unimportant or that it's my fault—the extreme (and unscientific) sizeism of the medical industry doesn't directly affect me. In myriad other ways, too, I walk into a system biased toward me—structurally designed to help people like me, staffed by people who view me as a sympathetic figure deserving of care, healing, dignity—and of life.

Then again, as a chronically ill person, I also walk into healthcare settings encumbered by others' conceptions of what my diagnosis means for who I am and how I can expect to live my life. What symptoms deserve attention, and what must simply be borne? What activities are open and closed to me? Which treatments are worth the hassle, pain, or expense, and which modalities matter? These are not always questions offered for me to answer about my body and my life, but ones doctors often answer themselves, according to their own assumptions. They're even questions that researchers and funders answer on my behalf when they deem chronic or rare illnesses less worthy of investigation than others.

This abstract conversation matters to our everyday lives because doctors have immense power over individuals' and groups' access to healing. Doctors have the authority to diagnose or dismiss, listen or lecture, experiment or empower, narrow horizons or expand options, and most importantly, to triage symptoms or treat whole people. Their decisions, and health insurance companies' willingness to pay for treatment, depend on scientists' ability to investigate and communicate their findings. And those scientists' careers, in turn, depend on research funding from pharmaceutical and biotechnology companies, and the priorities of nonprofits and universities. Every time you step into a doctor's office, you're relying on this ecosystem to help you access the most effective care.

You're also likely relying on many other forms of knowledge, though, that can make all the difference between illness and health but don't officially "count." Your own ability to access and describe your body's sensations matters to your treatment. Your intuition and your providers'—like Dr. Tim's gut instinct about autoimmunity and his half-retrieved memory from med school—could unravel mysteries the conscious mind can't dissect. Ask anyone who's spent multiple days in a hospital, and they're liable to tell you the emotional intelligence and practical experience of their nurses mattered more to them than the book-smart expertise of their doctors. And your caregivers' knowledge of environmental and public health, mental, emotional, and spiritual well-being, and respectful, open communication skills are all important for making sure your holistic needs are met.

Eastern and Indigenous medicines tend to intuit this, recognize the importance of people's physical, mental, emotional, and spiritual dimensions of health, and often treat multiple aspects of a person at once. But the American healthcare system only recognizes as "medicine" the narrowest of direct interventions. While my supplements, food costs, yoga classes, and alternative prophylactics have helped keep me off that thousands-of-dollars-per-week injection, I can't submit those costs to my health insurance company or even my tax-free, health-directed Flexible Spending Account. And of course, I'm lucky to have a doctor who takes those options seriously to begin with.

Our bodies—and the emotions that live in them—are sources of God-given wisdom. They respond with pleasure to flavorful foods, enjoyable movement, and time with loved ones; and they warn us with anxiety when danger is near, or with pain when we need to slow down and tend to them. Scientists are learning more and more about how we can work intelligently with them so that we're neither helpless victims of every feeling and sensation nor constantly repressing signals meant to support us.

We live as whole people. We experience illness as whole people. We heal as whole people. In fact, we do all these things, not only as individuals interconnected within ourselves, but also as beings who can't be cleanly divided from our families and communities, our experiences of privilege and oppression, or our places and environments. All these experiences and relationships constitute who we are in all our dimensions, not least in the physical domain. In other words, our physical health can depend upon attending to our own many dimensions, or to our contexts, as easily as it might depend upon something that might show up on a scan. But too often, when we walk into a doctor's office, we're reduced to a symptom or a body part—if we're lucky enough not to be reduced to stereotypes about our race, our gender, our size, or our sexuality.

––––––––

This medical saga wouldn't really be complete without some attention to what's not here. For every barrier to care and healing I faced, my privilege allowed me to skip, skirt, or hurdle another way our systems make people sick or prevent their access to healing.

I have excellent health insurance through my husband's job and even a diagnosis via the great healthcare I received as a child. I have a husband and parents who can (and do) support me when I need rest and/or care. I have an upper-middle-class White woman's familiarity with systems and cultures of bureaucracy, education and experience in convincing authority figures to take me seriously and do what I want, and the access and personal confidence to fire my doctor when they don't. I can afford all those treatment options I just noted that my insurance doesn't cover—a good investment, but still an expensive one. I have enough education to research my own condition and treatment without falling prey to a snake oil salesman. I can seek spiritual, emotional, and social healing without experiencing ongoing oppression due to my race, size, or sexuality. I even have the resources to attend to my environmental health. I was able to remediate the mold in my crawlspace, both because

I could afford to and because the house is mine—and if I had to, I could move.

As I watch this stack of privileges grow taller and taller, I'm also struck that these are all pretty basic human needs. So are things like mental health care, time to rest, resources for stress management, and safe, caring community. If all of these have been indispensable parts of my own healing, then they're not nice-to-have extras; they're things we all deserve access to.

Too often we blame people for getting sick—especially if they're poor or People of Color—when in fact they've never had access to the things they need to heal. The diet and wellness industries have convinced us that our individual health is under our own control. But as the pandemic has taught us, all of our health is deeply connected to each other's.

Likewise, we too often cast suspicion on ideas of "holistic health" because they're so often sold to us as individual "lifestyle" choices; but a truly holistic approach would recognize that we cannot be separated from our physical environments and social contexts. Attending to the whole person means attending to the communities and environments that they depend upon and contribute to. In other words, attending to our own health means concerning ourselves with our neighbors'. We might all get sick less often if all restaurant workers had paid sick leave. Healthcare costs would go down if everyone had access to the joyful movement, fresh food, and preventative care needed to prevent and manage chronic conditions before they became major emergencies.

When it comes to the healthcare system itself, many people in my country can't even imagine one based on sharing, but in fact our imaginations must be even more expansive than that if we want to live in a healthy country. We don't just need to be able to pay a doctor; we need doctors and researchers who actively resist their own biases and their fields'. We can't just recruit more nurses and home health aides when there's a shortage; we need to honor, and pay well for, their caring work just as we do for doctors' knowledge work. And we don't just need to find ways to pay for more and more drugs; we need structural supports—some as simple as sidewalks—to make basic human health needs like movement and sleep available to all. We need to recognize that public health is healthcare—much, much cheaper healthcare in the long run.

I'm tempted to find this line of thought discouraging. In the US COVID-19 response, we failed the biggest possible public health test: we failed to test and trace the disease; turned mask-wearing and vaccines into a political issue; cheered on our essential workers for about three weeks before we threw them back under the bus; and generally refused to face reality, accept responsibility, and care for our neighbors even after more than a million of them died. I believe that level of disconnection from our communities is about as sinful as a society can get.

But I've also known enough lifelong activists to recognize that cultural, large-scale change that seems inevitable in hindsight is glacially slow and uncertain when it's taking place. Besides our colossal failures, the United States's temporary expansions of federal anti-poverty measures are also historic, along with the massive campaign to offer vaccines to everyone for free. These programs have demonstrated just how possible it is to offer basic protections to everyone, and make our whole society safer as a result.

We are still deciding—as a country, and as individuals— who we want to be. The pandemic has changed things, and many of us intuit that we don't want to go back to the way things were. From small daily habits to major life decisions, we are looking for more life-giving and sustainable ways to be in the world. We want to reconnect with ourselves, earth, each other, and God—even if we hardly know how to say it, let alone do it. We're longing to make a place where we do better by one another—to act in alignment with the truth that we belong to each other.

It is time to listen closely to our pain, anger, and grief—and to our deep longings and great delights. So many days I am driven to distraction by my emotions, or caught up in today's "call to action" as a way of coping with them. But the way forward is not to forever swing between these two poles. It is to befriend my towering rages and unbidden tears, to sit with them long enough to hear what they are really telling me about myself and the world. It is to respect them enough to allow them to change not just my agenda for the afternoon, but the ways I look at my life and move about the world.

———

Tending to our own emotions doesn't seem like a meaning-ful solution to the injustices and failures of the US healthcare system; but in fact, slowing down to attend to our whole selves is cracking open a tiny window of space and time to redefine "health" and "care" for ourselves and embody a healing way of life toward others too. Anywhere we offer each other space to allow healing to take place, in safety, without rushing, can become a healing space in its own right. So often our hearts, bodies, and minds simply need rest and safe relationship where they can access their own wisdom and activate their own healing processes. We're not all doctors and therapists, but if we offered each other that kind of space, we could all become their accomplices.

Often, our first experiences in that work will be claiming that space for ourselves and within ourselves. When I first started telling folks that managing autoimmune disease was a part-time job, I wasn't crusading for anything. I was just sick of feeling vaguely ashamed of being unemployed, and tired of having to decide how much to reveal or hide about a thing that consumed my life. I still had plans to get back to a "regular" life and my normal breakneck pace. It took a few years of deliberately, defiantly carving out the space to respect my own healing process before I could even name that that was what I'd done—or notice that reclaiming a different way of life might do more good than returning to my old ambitions.

Like the sick woman reaching out to touch Jesus, we all have the choice to reclaim agency even while recognizing our own limitations and systemic constraints. Whether it is taking a single step to attend to our physical, mental, or spiritual health even amidst chronic illness, or a single step to mitigate our societal ills, we don't have to know everything or do everything before we can choose our own power. While we can't always choose what happens to us, or what options are available to us, we can almost always start with what *is* in our control. We can take a breath. We can take a walk. We can ask for help. When we are overwhelmed, we can remember that the only place to begin is with "the next right thing."

This is not to shout toxic positivity over grief about things that will never change and concerns about systemic issues. But it is to remind us that our media environments, our hyperextended social networks, and our Unprecedented Times are perfectly designed to mire us in overwhelm. Fear, rage, self-righteousness, and bad news constrict our focus to the headline in front of us. No company's business model is to empower us to get up from our seats and take action in our own neighborhoods.

In fact, it often seems that my most privileged friends are the most paralyzed by unjust systems and the uncertain future. We are so glutted with information, so used to neatly controlling our lives and futures, and so unacquainted with discomfort that bad news causes us to shut down. But when people who hold so much privilege give in to despair, we insult and abandon those who are likely to bear the great brunt of the problem—*and we disrespect ourselves.* We underestimate our basic human abilities to act, to connect with others, to care and create change.

While we have some duty to basically know what's going on and even to face it, to grieve it, we also bear responsibility for growing our own resilience in order to live amidst it and do our tiny part to repair it.

For so many of us, that means taking seriously our own need for healing and honoring our whole selves, even our wounds. This is how we show up to broader movements with our deepest integrity, our fullest gifts, and our hardest-won wisdom.

If each of us who reclaimed a healing life for ourselves only made it possible for one other person to begin imagining it, we might create change faster than we think. Our health and healthcare are failing even at the level of imagination, so for many of us, our changemaking must begin there. When we advocate for our integrated bodies and minds in exam rooms; when we preserve ancestral healing knowledge; when we shift our employment practices, church volunteer roles and expectations, or language around illness, we are already making change in the world out of our ability to imagine something better.

Each of these seemingly tiny changes matters to a wider movement to provide quality healthcare as a human right for all. We need to be well in order to advocate for change, implement it, and walk each other through its inevitable difficulties.

For those of us most thoroughly acquainted with the absurdities of the US health insurance system, it can be hard to avoid the conclusion that the endless paperwork, phone calls, appeals, inaccurate bills, and delayed care aren't mere inefficiencies, but actually function to keep sick people and our families too overwhelmed to advocate for change. When we're feeling our worst, we're also bogged down in administrative details, legal language, and intentionally opaque billing practices. Just when we are most desperate for rest, we are most deluged with demands on our resources to play a nonsensical game with an unfeeling opponent. The odds are only stacked more heavily against people who face discrimination due to race, gender identity, immigration status, or any number of factors at every turn.

This is when our (and our families' and friends') rage can be a gift to us. When we feel trapped into a fight, anger reminds us what we are fighting for and offers temporary fuel to counter despair. When we are tempted to doubt ourselves, anger insists: This should not be! Anger becomes a counterweight against fear.

Anger needs help from our other emotions and sources of wisdom. We can't use it to push away sadness and vulnerability, or as our only source of energy, without eventually succumbing to even more total burnout. We need each other's help to make wise choices and express our anger healthfully so that it doesn't become a source of harm. But even when anger is destructive, that doesn't mean it's all bad. There are beliefs and practices deciding who receives care, who benefits from it, and who doesn't, that need to be destroyed in order to grow something more beautiful in their place.

Jesus honored those who insisted that, as musician and activist Andre Henry sings, "it doesn't have to be this way." To pursue Wholeness within ourselves and for the wider world, we need to welcome and honor all the parts of ourselves—despite what we've been told to scorn, shame, or hide. This is healing that grows and lasts.

PART III

5

THE ECONOMY AND OTHER CONVENIENT FICTIONS

Before my Behçet's returned, I would have told you God loves everyone, even and especially sick people, and that illness is no one's fault. As months went by, though, my conviction began to erode. I couldn't ride my bike anymore; fatigue pressed me to the bed; I came to dread sex as much as I wanted it. I slowly let go of the fantasy that this would all be over in a few weeks and I'd be back to interval training in no time. Without a job, a functioning body, or the ability to care for my family, what was God expecting me to *do*?

To some the answer might have been obvious: sick people pray for healing. Certainly, when a symptom grew intolerable, I prayed the flare would abate. I prayed for healing as a child too, but perhaps as much because I was "supposed" to as anything else. I did want to be well; I'd just never been convinced God "gave" me this disease so he could take it away.

While I didn't pray often for miraculous healing, I did pray I'd be able to do all the things I thought I was supposed to do. There was a list, a get-to-know-people-and-contribute-to-your-new-community list in my head telling me how to be a Good Person in Charleston. I needed to be volunteering, networking and socializing, getting involved with a church, exploring and learning our new town. These, I knew, were things God would have me do. God doesn't call people to move to new towns and lie prone on their couches, right?

As the question occurred to me, I admitted there was no reason God couldn't do that . . .

But surely God wouldn't call *me* to do such a thing?

God knew, you see, that I was special. Teachers had told me I was the star of every classroom and activity from age five on up. I was destined for greatness; this is what you learn in the suburbs, in advanced classes, in marching band leadership training, and especially in an evangelical pew. You learn your life is a "special mission" to bring glory to God, probably by adopting ten children or being the next Billy Graham, or making exorbitant amounts of money and giving a comfortable chunk away.

As I continued asking the same question and avoiding the same answer, it occurred to me that if our achievements are what matter, I, on my couch, was probably bringing less glory to God than my puppy, Miya, who at least brought joy to everyone everywhere she went. I developed a bit of jealousy toward the dog. Was it my new vocation to act as personal assistant to her?

Lonely, aimless, and suffering, I'd periodically come to the end of my question-prayers and finally hurl that one at God like an adolescent checkmate: *Did you bring me here to Charleston just to rescue this dog?*

When I heard anything back, it was only this:

What if such a thing did bring me pleasure? Would that be so bad?

I puzzled and raged like some sort of Chronic Illness Grinch. OF COURSE it would be so bad. It was a waste of my enormous potential! And people need to fill our days with more than books. And we need to feel important. And the dog—however delightful she may be—it's not like she was preventing hunger and homelessness here! All she did was love people unconditionally. And invite them into a spirit of play. And ask us to be in the moment with her. And live with a sense of expectancy that everyone loved her. And greet the mundane with wonder and delight.

And what if, what if, what if such things did bring God pleasure?

What if *I*, by simply existing as myself, made God's world a better place, like Miya did to mine?

What if my life story didn't have to be about the impact I made—the stuff I do, move, acquire, build—but about my own simple, still being?

Could it even be that, by learning to be still, I began to witness the gentle, slow, incremental ways the world reshapes around my still presence to it?

YES! GOT IT! Stillness. Excellent! My vocation as a sick person must be to master the art of meditation. I would become the very best at stillness. Then, everyone around me would inevitably become stiller and wiser because I was just that good at being still.

———

Looking back, I didn't know how to do anything, including have a chronic illness, without trying to achieve perfection at it. I didn't have an idea what a vocation might be if it wasn't a calling to be the very best at something. I couldn't conceive of my own value or the value of stillness if it didn't change the world and make me famous (or at least well-liked).

My doctor kept telling me I needed to lower my stress levels. This, of course, sounded positively immoral. What is a modern feminist without busyness; a young, smart college grad without obsessive ambition; an activist without chronic overwork and extreme political anxiety? "No one can completely eliminate stress from their lives," stress-reduction-advice counseled, and I nodded my vigorous agreement. I tried to ignore the fact that they meant to say *certain stressors are inevitable*, which I merely took as an excuse not to deal with my stressors at all. I didn't know who I was without them.

The truth is, I needed my stress to prove I was doing the best I could. Everyone around me was so stressed, it would feel entitled to presume to exempt myself. Books and websites suggested some ways to manage stress, and I much preferred to add these to my miles-long to-do list than to actually let go of any of my activities, anxieties, expectations, or achievements.

But the more months went by, the more I learned about stress, and the more stubbornly my hormone levels loitered in the doldrums. As my doctor explained my lab panels to me, it seemed like every other word she uttered was "stress." Chronic stress shortens telomeres, the protective structures at the end of a chromosome whose deterioration causes aging. Chronic stress increases blood pressure, suppresses the immune system, and causes inflammation—the core issue from which all my other issues stemmed.

The way our society organizes our days and our lives leaves our bodies far too often in fight-or-flight mode. Chemically, we are unable to distinguish between a tiger attack and the low-level panic of an average day commuting, playing for power at work, rushing to meet deadlines, nearly missing a child's soccer game, checking the bank account and feeling the heart rate spike. We're flooded with hormones meant to shift our bodies from their normal activities into emergency mode. But emergency mode itself becomes dangerous when we spend all our time there; it interrupts our bodies' other functions and its chemical by-products overwhelm our systems. Stress wears down the body as thoroughly and predictably as racing wears down a stock car.

After enough time under this onslaught, my immune system and its haywire hormones responded. Pushed beyond a breaking point and unable to process the situation, it lashed out at the phantom threat unbalancing the body—swinging, missing, and damaging the body itself in the process. The immune system under sustained stress acts like most people do under stress: doing its best under an extreme overload, it actually creates a spiral of destruction.

Compared to the earlier days when I worked through grad school as a catering server, then planned a wedding and a cross-country move, I hardly *felt* stressed, I protested; but that wasn't exactly true. No, I didn't struggle to complete all my assignments or pay my rent, but I did cram my life full of events and activities in an attempt to feel significant, productive, connected. I worried about my career and I worried about the state of the country. I got a part-time job at a new church plant. I wrote every morning. I joined the Poor People's Campaign. I put my guest bedroom on Airbnb. I traveled an average of twice a month for work, writing, family. I cooked and cleaned and maintained our family's social calendar.

I did this all in an attempt to fulfill perceived expectations of what it meant to be productive, responsible, generous, worthy, good. Then I decided I wasn't making impressive enough progress on a career, so I decided to start a business. I made a plan and pursued it at full steam for a few weeks, until fatigue forced me to admit that my body and I were currently not business-owner material—not without quitting absolutely everything else.

It wasn't until a couple of weeks after I "postponed" the business that I really recognized the absurdity of trying to do all this at once. At one point, so many people had affirmed my business idea that it seemed crazy not to try while I was young, childless, in possession of some cash. Now I wondered what else might actually be better left undone.

———

For so long I'd refused to consider that I was no longer tough, no longer strong, that all my discipline and will no longer counted for anything. Some sweet friend will object that they did count, that I am mentally tougher and braver than ever before! But that doesn't ring true to me. I think I was toughest when I went through all this as a nine-year-old.

The truth is, my default reaction to adversity was to power through, but I eventually had to acknowledge that there are times when working harder and fighting more will only make us weaker. My intense workouts and self-improvement projects had actively contributed to the breakdown of my body. Fragility and fussiness were my companions now. At some point, denying it in the name of "toughness" would only make me a stooge.

Maybe my needs for rest and accommodation weren't my biggest obstacles; maybe my own contempt for fragility was. To me every weakness and vulnerability was a failure—something to be overcome. But when you've pushed a system past its breaking point, the old rules no longer apply. Reliable tactics don't lead to the same outcomes anymore. Working harder—despising my fragility and believing I could eradicate it—only made it more evident. After twenty-six years of constant self-improvement, I could no longer get better.

To my ears there is still no way to say that I "accepted my weakness" without sounding as though I merely *succumbed.* But could it be that acceptance is its own way of choosing, of claiming agency? Can someone be fragile *and* resilient? Needy and needed?

We often insist upon calling survivors of illness "fighters." Surely many of them are. But some of us are not. Some of us have had enough of internal battling. Some of us are not fighters of disease but students of it. Some of us are gatherers of the weak. Some of us are witnesses and chroniclers. Some of us are artists.

When I had the courage to let go of despising my own weakness, suddenly there was room for tenderness to flood in. Fragility and vulnerability didn't have to be places of hatred, fear, and despair; instead, they began to call me not only into acceptance and kindness, but even into possibility.

Outside of humanity, we hold admiration for plenty of fragile things: flower petals and butterflies, complex clockworks and ancient works of art. Delicacy can be a marker of beauty and of a satisfying sort of complexity—a call for protection and care that is more awe-filled than burdensome. What more could I want from (and for) my body?

Even more importantly, relinquishing my ability to be strong and "whole" on my own revealed that ability had always been an illusion anyway. We are not units meant to function on our own. Our weaknesses bind us to one another in ways that are not shameful but reveal and magnify each other's beauty.

———

As I flipped through the files of my life, wondering what to slow down on and what to toss completely, it was the activist in me who clung most tightly to all her imagined obligations. I knew that if I set down my picket sign I would collapse on the sidewalk in long-delayed tears. My striving busyness was what allowed me to assiduously avoid both grief for the world and frustration at it. I didn't know how to just *be* with a world hurting due to injustice without my indignation and my plans to fix it. Even knowing the cost to my body, I struggled to imagine that I could be allowed or invited to rest while so many others have no choice but to pay for their lives in the currency of stress.

How many of the impoverished people I'd known who lived in constant pain were dying of forever being forced to fight or flee—of encountering their own lives as enemies? I was falling apart from stress without multiple jobs, children, relying on faulty public transit or substandard housing, the unnecessary paperwork and office visits of welfare, over-policing, impossible financial choices, racial or other discrimination, and the constant nagging threat that one unpreventable emergency could cause utter disaster. In this context, I often couldn't tell whether my own pain could really mean that I truly required radical rest, or if its urgent throb was calling me into even deeper solidarity with other people in pain.

I also couldn't access a world where there might be more than one answer. It took a long time to wonder where I absorbed the idea that it was a binary choice.

Beneath my many layers of anxiety about vocation lay another struggle: the seemingly impossible demand to accept that I am disabled. Today, in the five-plus years since I was totally stuck on the couch, most of my symptoms have abated most of the time, but I still live every day with a limited reserve of energy. I've experienced healing, but I continue to be unable to work full-time without risking my health, and potentially my life. The societal attitude that people with "comorbidities" are expendable in the context of COVID-19 has further sidelined me from the nondisabled world.

These facts being what they may, it took all five of those years—until I was partway through writing this book—before I actually uttered that sentence: *I am disabled.* In the summer of 2021, I wrote in my journal:

> I am still coming to terms with how unreachable the "normal" world is for me. I've had to reimagine my world so many times: a world with arthritic fingers and without rock climbing, a world with a delicate digestive system and without bread baking, a world with fatigue and without a nice, office-y career.
>
> I am writing from the outside. I have had to make my home in a place I once considered an unfortunate pit stop; a place where chronic illness is, in fact, perennially persistent, a country on a shifting borderland where "chronically ill" meets "disabled." I'm still trying to look clearly at my temporary shelters and understand how they are to become permanent. I still don't know how to introduce myself as a citizen of this place.

Even if I were magically cured tomorrow, I don't think I'd be able to return to my old land either. So many things I used to expect from myself and others now seem not only unattainable, but actually ill-advised.

As I write in these strange pandemic months, I'm keenly aware of how many others feel similarly. What *were* we even doing before, and why did it feel so inevitable back then? How much of it can we possibly return to on this changed and fragile planet?

Theologian Nancy L. Eiesland describes the wisdom found in this experience of disability: "Ordinary lives incorporate contingency and difficulty . . . Limits are real human facts and . . . heroism cannot eliminate some limits."

Yet, while we embody this wisdom that applies to everyone, disabled people also differ from nondisabled people in that our sometimes-difficult "ordinary lives" are made more difficult by structural barriers and societal stigmas. No longer able to work full-time, I don't count in much of the political talk of "the economy"—or in the eyes of many of the people I meet. Unable to risk a COVID-19 infection, I'm stranded outside the life that has resumed for so many nondisabled others.

Eiesland names my experience coming to terms with the word "disabled" in a single sentence: "Our struggle against the discrimination that is pervasive within the church and society [is] part of the work of coming to our bodies." Pursuing a right relationship of Wholeness with my body meant continuing to recognize how her experience is shaped not only by a misogynist, but also an ableist world—and how that experience is shared by others.

My very first draft of this book made no mention of ableism. It was easier to talk about things that affected other people, even my own sins, than to really face the way other people devalue and discard *me*. I would rather tell a story about "exploiting myself" than face the other half of the same story. If I hadn't been married to someone with a well-paying job, the US disability systems would have forced me into severe poverty—or I would have had to continue working full-time through fatigue, with no energy available for anything else, including healing.

As it is, though I have a little writing work, my husband is basically my patron. I can heal, create, organize and protest, and care for others because I am dependent on him. I hear what others really think of people like me when they talk about policies like universal basic income or "Medicare for All" as preposterous fairytales. They think my life of basic security—the environment that has allowed me to live without constant pain—is a lucky jackpot at best, lazy and immoral at worst. They believe people like me deserve to wear ourselves down to nubs in order to live, until finally one day we are gone—which is exactly what happens every day to those who face poverty, medical discrimination, and medical debt.

I also struggled to see myself as disabled because I clung to the illusion that I *was* able, that my life and my body could still "count" in the eyes of others. Most of us are afraid to talk about ableism. We don't want to acknowledge how close we all are to "losing everything"—not necessarily because life with a disability is inherently bad, but because our society is all too willing to *take* everything from disabled people. Life with a disability is different, but for many disabled people, our bodies are simply our bodies and our lives are simply our lives. We don't experience ourselves as tragedies, obstacles, or non-entities, but nondisabled people fear becoming like us because *they* see us that way.

We're also afraid to confront our own ableism because disability access upends our national religion of efficiency. If we took everyone's needs seriously, it would cost time and resources. Better, we assume, to relegate lack of access to the category of "personal problems" or even collateral damage than to expend limited resources growing the hospitality and dignity of our environments.

This misunderstanding of efficiency is also why I refuse to oppose small-scale transformation against widespread, systemic change. My earlier, rather arbitrary opposition between *resting* and *acting* in solidarity with others came to seem like a foreign relic of my "old land." That dichotomy is based on a single model of linear, unending, machine-like, measurable "progress" that bears little resemblance to the patterns we find in nature—or in ourselves. If overlooked actions of care, writing and making art, learning to heal, or creating community aren't allowed to count as activism, then many of my disabled friends and I can never belong.

Instead, in meetings and projects, I learned to make humbler promises: I will do what I can; I will ask for help when I need it; I will find a way to show up even if it requires a little creativity. These habits contributed to a bolder promise: a promise to *stay.* In organizing my work so I could do it sustainably, I committed not to checking the right number of tasks off a list, but to participating in steady, deep-rooted transformation over time—rather than lurching, surface-level change on a timeline of false urgency. I couldn't always "serve the world" with any specific promises of great efficiency or productivity, but I could serve a few people through friendship, or serve an organization by doing administrative tasks that felt piddly, or serve my church by asking good questions.

These types of service were far from the version of leadership I'd grown up believing myself to be destined for. I was no longer the person working the hardest, having a plan, making things happen, casting a great vision, fixing a big problem, or making sure everyone "got things right." Having remembered the word "no," I no longer had a hand in ten different projects either. I was the person showing up to one place unnoticed, taking direction, tending to what others had grown, having to trust someone else's leadership, learning with difficulty to do what Mother Teresa called "small things with great love."

Disabled people can and *must* lead businesses, churches, and organizations. But as a person who had previously lived with so much privilege, I had much more to learn from the humble practice of showing up to do mundane tasks than from gaining yet more "experience" finding yet another leadership position. I discovered the power of faithfulness, tending to the same small things over and over, to matter to the world and to transform *me.* From my place outside the "norm," I learned what it was like for my limited body, my limited life, and my limited contributions to be overlooked—and that, painful and unfair as it was, I also wouldn't die from lack of recognition.

And I learned a more subtle art of discernment. Earlier in life, I'd thought of "vocational discernment" as deciding which path I would take to greatness. I surmised that it involved lots of prayer, great lightning bolts of revelation, hard work and adventures, and being rewarded with success and satisfaction. Now I had to carefully discern questions like, *Will this one-hour-a-month task fit into my limited number of "productive" hours per month?* It involved a whole matrix of follow-up questions that I'd rarely been encouraged to ask about acts of service. Did I even *want* to do the thing? Would it help me build relationships or trust with a community of people? Would it take time away from things I needed to do to care for myself? Did the mission or purpose

I was serving make my heart sing with joy? *Was this really mine to do?*

Despite my frustration at my disease, other days it comes as an exquisite relief to have a name for living conscientiously with my own limits. The more I embrace my enforced simplicity, the more I wonder at the frantic paces of others. I've become greedy for margin, and baffled by a culture that almost treats it with suspicion or disdain.

The further removed I become from my burnout life, the more I find myself—in otherwise ordinary moments— confused and out of place in my burnout world. My body relentlessly presses the same question onto me: How much of this activity is truly necessary? It seems increasingly strange that this question is so rarely asked in the wider world.

There was no definitive moment when I escaped my fear that without work, busyness, and stress I would no longer matter—it's been a slow process that may never end. I still rage some days against my own limits, which have become as immediate and immovable as the walls containing my home. I can no longer "be anything I want to be," but I'm not sure I could do that before when I believed it either. All our choices close off other possibilities; all our most sacred priorities come with real costs.

———

The evidence that Jesus had really risen from the dead was the evidence that he'd been overtaken and killed. The wisdom of disability lives in God's body too.

"Although the doors were shut, Jesus came and stood among them and said, 'Peace be with you.' Then he said to Thomas, 'Put your finger here and see my hands. Reach out

your hand and put it in my side. Do not doubt but believe'"
(John 20:26–27 NRSV). In a redeemed body, on the other
side of death, still he bore his wounds. Still his body did
not conform to anyone else's expectations of power; still it
might even have offended or disgusted. But this was the evidence. This was the truth of himself, presented to seal his
reunion with his friends. This was the way the risen Lord
went about the world.

Eiesland calls this Jesus a *survivor.* He has walked into the
worst of empire, been undone by the breaking of Wholeness
between him and his people, between him and his friends,
and finally the violation of his bodily integrity—through to
the other side. It's made him neither helpless and pitiable,
nor unequivocally "stronger." Instead, his experience of
isolation and violence remains a part of him, and one his
friends must encounter in order to know and worship him.

Jesus shows us that a "healthy" or "whole" or redeemed
body is not one without fissure, not an independent, unac-
commodated one, not one that makes other people feel comfortable. It is one that includes *itself*, owns its own history
of exclusion and suffering, and shows up to social space a
survivor of these things. This body, to borrow Sonya Renee
Taylor's phrasing, "is not an apology." Instead, Jesus asks his
friends to see and to touch his wounds.

Jesus's survivor's body mediates God to the world. For
Eiesland, "The disabled God embodies the ability to see
clearly the complexity and the 'mixed blessing' of life and
bodies, without living in despair." This is the evidence: not
beauty, ability, or strength, but a body broken *and* whole,
offered yet again to the embrace of his friends.

———

Now that I live with a lot less margin, I still struggle when I can't point to all the ways I'm laboring or sacrificing to make the world a better place. It's very well to reject the idea that our value lies in our labor, but that doesn't diminish the desire most adults I know have *to be useful*, to at least occasionally make some contribution to others' lives. For some of my disabled friends and me, this is a great, perhaps an existential, struggle.

My hunch is that the real root of our struggle isn't that we never do anything for anyone. It's that we were taught from early ages that the kinds of contributions we can make don't "count." We may not be able to go to a full-time job, but we may be able to offer hospitality, be present in a space, pray, tend land, pursue artistic and creative endeavors, listen to people, get friends to their doctors' appointments, offer a different perspective to an organization, do independent reading and research, and engage in the very serious intensive work of perpetually healing.

Few people get paid to do these things, so they're all culturally presumed to fall under "extracurriculars" for adults. But in reality, these activities constitute the threads that invisibly hold the world together. Our failure to provide for the people who do them is a failure to value them appropriately. They represent spiritual, relational, mental, and creative labor that nondisabled people too often neglect to name as such. And in so doing, they neglect invisible, essential maintenance for the whole web of life.

Our empire of capitalism is obsessed with growth, with building new things and expanding old ones; we laud (and pay for) anything that can be called "pioneering." But the US pioneers who saw themselves as "making something" of empty space were actually destroyers of ecosystems and civilizations. They failed (often rather deliberately) to see the value of Indigenous ecosystem management, communities, and spiritualities, or of communities of plants, animals, and soil and the work they do.

The systems and cultures we've inherited from those pioneers continue to erase, discount, and devalue work of maintenance, tending, and relating, especially when it is done by women, People of Color, and disabled people, among others. We may struggle even to recognize these skilled, necessary, and resource-intensive activities as "work." But—as women are so subtly and deftly trained from birth to know—nothing gets done if no one cleans the coffeepot, smooths over hurt feelings after a meeting, watches the children, waters the plants, remembers to buy toilet paper, and orders cake for Chad's birthday.

When we experience comfort, care, camaraderie, security, and joy in our businesses, churches, or organizations, we often attribute it to an amorphous "sense of community" or to a manager's skill. But these qualities don't just appear; they are created. They are the sum of those "little" tasks that are so often rendered invisible. Likewise, when an organization appears to be slowly disintegrating with no discernible cause, we are often struggling to name an absence of these sustaining qualities and the conditions that create them.

Good care isn't controlling; it's listening. Good care doesn't exploit; it empowers. Good care takes place in relationships of reciprocity. Good care is massively creative, but because the creation is sometimes invisible (or gets composted), it is overlooked in our consumerist society. If we are trying to dismantle systems and cultures of domination, maybe honoring the works of maintenance, tending, healing, and accompaniment would get us farther than we think.

Jesus's wounded hands sanctify the vocation of survival. When women, disabled folks, and other marginalized people care for each other, we are doing the healing work of God. When we invite our whole, wounded, or rejected selves into that work, we are restoring Wholeness within ourselves and offering right relationship with us to the world. When we help each other survive and thrive, we are subverting the empire that would prefer to leave us behind.

Caring and relational work may be repetitive and it may go unseen, but it is not lesser work. Sometimes the very best teacher and the most supportive action is a simple act of care, undertaken with sensitivity, in service of solidarity.

Many marginalized communities have developed a particular genius for creating networks of mutual aid—of care. The term "mutual aid" gained popularity during the early days of COVID-19 as a way of talking about any community effort to respond dynamically to the many crises at hand. But the phrase has a long history of very specific use among minoritized people and activists: It's meant to refer to projects and organizations that intentionally subvert the traditional power dynamics of "charity," where a giver is assumed to have some status over, or hold some debt from, a receiver. Mutual aid efforts emphasize structures and cultures that encourage reciprocity, seek equity, and build community and political power among people who understand themselves as both givers and receivers.

Some of these are formal organizations, and some primarily distribute funds, but they are often inspired by informal networks of people who simply take care of each other to survive. For many poor and houseless people, LGBTQIA+

chosen families, Black and Brown neighborhoods, and patient advocacy groups and networks of disabled friends, this is simply a way of life.

As COVID-19 lingers, we continue to see how vital caring roles are in our society—from nursing home workers to hospital chaplains to mother-ers—but we remain at a loss for how to properly value the labor of tending to the invaluable.

What would happen if we made a discipline of naming and celebrating the labor people undertake to care for themselves or others; to journey into the wilds of the creative realm; to offer emotional or practical support to others; to be holistically and spiritually present to the world; or to be faithful to repetitive tasks of maintenance? Would we start to break down the false construct that "work" only pertains to what is profitable?

Too many of us have learned to equate "being useful" with being used. We think work is supposed to be difficult and deadlined. But what if we practiced luxuriating in the usefulness of labor that comes easily to us, that connects us to others, that creates something superfluous, that has the repetitive rhythm of prayer?

It's a tool of White-cis-hetero-male supremacy to erase and dismiss those acts. Let's start naming them and valuing them: in our movements, our job descriptions, our wage scales.

This is not a sidestep or an "answer" to the grief of losing activities, jobs, or dreams when we become disabled. But it is a rebuke to the silence that falls when we finally whisper to someone, *I just want to be useful again.*

I don't believe that God uses people. I don't believe, either, that God dangles promises of holiness or justice in front of us so that we'll exploit and abuse ourselves. Instead,

God co-creates and co-labors with us, and God does so most insistently, most powerfully when our creation and labor are slow, invisible, and full of great love. Such is the work of our care, the gift to the world of our rest, the deeply necessary contributions of our art, our prayer, our witness to lives on the margins. Here is work so weighty and so joyful that God insists on doing it by our side.

6

HEALING IS PRICELESS

In 2021, when I began writing this book, the world was in as much disarray as ever. California was decimated by wildfires, Louisiana and Tennessee by storms. The Taliban retook Afghanistan. My friends were organizing to lobby the state legislature about education and COVID-19. People were scared. People had real, urgent needs.

Every day, I got up and wrote words and took care of myself.

I'd take a walk and do yoga. I cooked for myself. I cleaned my house to keep my own spirits up. I scheduled calls and dates with friends. I called this success.

For most of my adult life, I considered every one of those tasks "personal time" and tried to cram them in between work, volunteering, writing, and trying to comprehend the entire world and what to do about it. Now, they consumed my days. I'd decided to live as if this work of writing was work enough; as if my own sacred being was worth stewarding well—even in the midst of tragedy and chaos.

I instinctively reach for a defense of my limited "productivity" while the world is so full of need. I could tell you about the exact cytokines the body produces in response to chronic stress, which have been directly linked to increased severity of my particular disease. Or I could simply say I'd decided to experimentally confirm my sneaking suspicion that I feel better physically when I am happier. Or should I tell you that we wanted a baby, and I was supposed to reduce stress for that reason too?

In the end, my only "defense" is an intuition: that I really must unhook from the belief that the world will improve in proportion to my productivity, that oh-so-much depends on me at all times. I am trying to resist the internal need to defend my rest at all.

As my experiment unfolded, I was surprised to find how quickly and naturally my determined *lack* of activity actually affected the world. I invited my neighbor to join me for yoga in my yard, bringing respite to her weeks of tending to students, parents, and teachers. I had time in an afternoon to bring some tea along to another friend in the midst of important leadership work. A third friend sat on my porch on a different morning reciting a litany of tasks and projects she wished she could cancel, "but things still have to happen," she sighed with bone-deep weariness. I caught her eye. "Do they?" I said, trying to be gentle. "What if, in the midst of an ongoing global emergency, nothing *has* to happen besides surviving?"

"*No one* has margin, *everyone* is in despair," headlines and friends said alike. For so many years I'd taken statements like this to mean that *I* don't "deserve" to be the exception. When so many people have no choice but to be under constant stress, how could I sit back? How did I dare to pursue peacefulness?

Trying it now, for the first time in my life, I quickly began to wonder why I thought I deserved to be so self-importantly busy and constantly off-kilter all the time. Now that I was paying attention to the people and needs right in front of me—starting with my own—I found I had not retreated from the rest of the world at all, but had *more* resources available to take exquisite care of those right around me who so deeply needed and deserved it.

With or without chronic illness, we all have limitations and needs. But when circumstances seem dire, when we are constantly encouraged to continue dividing our attention, when we're lulled by the false promise of constant "progress" and the subtle threat that rest equals failure, we view our limitations as enemies. Underneath our frustration, fear, or shame about our limits lies the seductive, if absurd, lure of the limitless life. And why shouldn't it? We've been discipled by extractive capitalism in the false gospel of limitless growth.

Oddly, though, it's the business and "productivity" worlds where the trend is to acknowledge and accept limits. The principle of essentialism reminds us that when we spread our ambitions too thin, we actually fail to make progress on any of our goals. Better to choose one or two, focus, and concentrate our limited energy in the direction that's most important and most suited to our own strengths.

But we fear saying "no." We forget to count the costs of our inner work, our caring work, our healing work. We pile on tasks, try to keep up with the hourly news, and say yes to one more invitation, because it seems like we "should." Because everyone else looks like they're keeping up. Because a constant harrying *not enough* whispers in our ear.

That's how the ableism in our culture—the belief that our hustle will prove our worth, busyness as a badge of honor, the expectation that we'll demonstrate our commitment to something by doing more and more—hurts us all. Even when we seem to be managing our overtaxed lifestyles, we're half-assing important tasks, half-paying-attention to important relationships, and half-aware of whether the things we're doing are really ours to do at all. Whether intentional or not, keeping us busy and stressed is a great strategy for distracting us from participating in our democracy, building resilient communities of solidarity, or pursuing groundedness and peace—and a great strategy for selling us stuff. Meanwhile—sick or not—our bodies under stress are slowly wearing down.

Of all the issues in this book that affect privileged and oppressed people differently, "the economy" seems like the one that would most obviously have vastly different consequences for different people. But while our capitalist economy serves to make some people very poor and others very rich, it also creates a culture where almost *all* of us experience more stress and isolation than ever before. For low-wage workers, it might be imposed by "just-in-time" scheduling at an hourly job and the emotional toll of financial precarity, while wealthy people are likely to work upwards of sixty hours a week as a job requirement and a status symbol. Both situations can chronically put the body under more strain than it can handle. However, one group has the resources to support their bodies and find ways to cope; the less-resourced group is simply left to manage amidst a vortex of other disadvantages.

"The economy"—our current system of neoliberal capitalism whose religion is faith in the "invisible hand" of the market—so thoroughly organizes our politics and our lives that we *all* live to some degree by its rhythms and rules. From that religion we learn that our value is in our productivity, our status or belonging hinges on our consumption, and our future depends solely on ourselves and our own effort in competition with others. We also learn to model our creative lives, our churches, and our relationships with ourselves on "successful" businesses and economies: expecting constant, linear growth, at all times, forever. These assumptions about work and worth seep into our interactions with ourselves and others, into our businesses and organizations, into our schools and relationships with our children. Rich or poor, we rarely even question the assumption that, unless we're willing and able to work harder than the person next to us, we're not worthy to have the resources to live or a sense of purpose in life.

Consumption becomes the soother of exhaustion and anxiety, and the proof to ourselves and the world that we're successful, we're worthy, and we belong. We've all been so efficiently trained into doing and having (or giving and being) more, more, more, that we no longer have a reference point for *enough*. We no longer have any inkling that the more, more, more must come from somewhere. We draw incessantly from reserves—of oil, of forest, of our own bodies' energy—that we don't actually have. And every catastrophe is inviting us to recognize those limits. Reality will continue to crash in on us until we finally submit to reality.

The insistence by research that the body isn't designed to live this way finally forced me to consider that maybe stress isn't the price of admission to adulthood. It's not virtuous to be overwhelmed by your life and oppressed by your schedule. It may be seasonally necessary, but those seasons aren't supposed to be the norm. When they were, I ended up spreading myself too thin until I finally pulled myself apart.

———————

Of course, those most negatively affected by our culture's outsized expectations are those with the least choice in the matter. If you're working three minimum wage jobs just to keep your lights on, you can philosophize (or be sick) all you want, but the rent will not go down. Your inhumane schedule isn't a mental block; it's the result of massive income inequality and a social safety net full of barbs and holes.

Still, at the heart of US policy debates on poverty thrums the more-more-more anthem of America. We both idolize hard work and denigrate "unskilled labor" as an excuse for keeping our essential workers in dire poverty. We dangle improbable success stories as judgments on those who hit too many roadblocks to escape a system designed to trap them. Insidiously, middle- and upper-class Americans can be convinced to believe that our own (college-educated, essential-worker-facilitated) "hard work" entitles us to what we have. Some part of us is afraid to slow down purely because we'd then lose our flimsy excuse not to look inequality in the face. If we admitted that there might be plenty of space and resources available in our own lives, we might need to pay more attention to the distribution of plenty in the rest of our big, wealthy, overstimulated country.

It's not a high bar, in the wealthiest country in the world, to claim that everyone should have *enough*: enough to eat, enough to afford rent, access to healthcare and education. For all our political talk of "the economy," it seems reasonable to expect everyone to benefit from its workings. But even though politicians use "the economy" as shorthand for "everyone's well-being," it doesn't actually translate that way. When huge swaths of people can't earn enough to live, the economy is not serving them. If the rest of us are burning ourselves out on its behalf, it's not serving us either.

The good and beautiful news is that if we put a higher value on margin—recognized the abundance around us—rediscovered *enough*—middle-class people might also feel less threatened by slightly higher taxes or marginally higher prices. It's only the more-more-more mindset, and that tattered social safety net, that make us think we need rock-bottom prices to afford to live well, or that poverty relief programs don't benefit us by making our whole community healthier.

Every time policy ideas come up for reducing poverty, from the local level to the national or even global, we have an opportunity to begin creating a world where fewer of our neighbors are living in fight-or-flight mode. We are imagining the beginnings of a humane and healing economy. If it would require us to make less war or pay more taxes, maybe those could be healing practices too. Maybe our immune systems, our social fabric, and our planet have had *enough* of stress, strain, and growth-at-all-costs.

Likewise, every time we choose *enough* over more-more-more, we enact a tiny revolt against the idol-worship of productivity and the economy. When we practice discernment to narrow down our commitments, find creative ways to share, or coach our kids or ourselves in the way of good enough, we push back against the anxiety and exhaustion of the never-enough mindset. And we begin to teach our bodies, and maybe our neighbors, that they are safe with us.

When it comes to stress, some of us have the freedom to "simplify our lives" rather straightforwardly, by changing our schedules or our spending habits. But for many of us, it is paradoxically complicated at first. There's the money, ambition, and purpose we draw from our careers and our consumer habits, or the caring responsibilities we can't just cut loose because they're stressful. Or there's the chronic illness—the doctor's appointments, self-advocacy, weird drugs, weird foods, bills, and frayed social networks just when symptoms zap all energy for those things.

Whether we want to simplify for our own bodies, for our minds, for the world, or all of the above, it's too easy to turn "simplifying" into yet another urgent project. Ever set a deadline to KonMari your entire house in hopes that total peace would fall upon your home by next Tuesday? We forget how to have a goal without a long to-do list, deadlines, and shopping lists that paradoxically land us right back where we started—only adding to our sense of overwhelm and falling "behind."

The desire to simplify can be an invitation to try another way of making change. After all, "a simple life" looks different for different people at different times and places. We'll always be relearning and reevaluating what it means to us. There's freedom in letting a process be a process—in letting something unfold. Saying "no" to one thing on our schedule and paying close attention to how that makes us feel might lead to far more lasting change than rage-quitting everything that used to bring joy or implementing a complex system of productivity and time hacks.

In the past, I've constructed plenty of those grandiose plans and projects to fix my life. Especially when the change I want to make is driven by necessity or by my deeply held values, it's easy for me to saddle the process with untenable urgency, perfectionism, and painful self-criticism. But I am learning that the gracious way, the slow-and-steady way, the sense of humor way, is also a way forward.

Often, with little energy and big needs, it's been the only way forward available to me. Disease and disability are slowly teaching me the shape of *enough*. *Enough* sleep, *enough* activity, the self-kind way of *good enough.*

———

"Good enough" wasn't always a phrase in my vocabulary. Some of my perfectionistic and overachieving habits are my own innate tendencies, but as I've tried to unlearn my stressed-out, burned-out lifestyle, I've noticed just how deeply those same tendencies run in the church culture I grew up in. It's easy for me to rail against capitalism as the engine of our attitudes of scarcity and our obsession with "productivity." I've never been one to chase a massive salary or fancy title, and still these attitudes and obsessions are as deeply ingrained in me as in anyone else.

Too many churches, nonprofits, and activist movements have claimed to reject the cruelties of capitalism while clinging fiercely to some of its most dehumanizing habits. We glorify overwork and lack of pacing. We model our organizations on businesses that pursue unlimited growth rather than on nature's cyclical seasons.

Many of us are locked in battles against systems and cultures of domination that turn out to be the wrong battles. Sometimes we are calling each other to action long before we know what the action is or whether it is really ours to take.

We demand each other's labor as if it could prove our love. I'm guilty of clamoring to be right, without humbly seeking to be in right relationship. We imply to people that they can never be good enough, projecting an image of some sort of self-improvement league when really we're a roomful of wounded underdogs. We are greedy for external proof of our own significance, for praise, for an intoxicating sense of righteousness, and we turn our pursuits of justice into joyless, exhausting endeavors.

The truth is, capitalism might have shaped the systems that taught me that "personal time" mattered less than "productivity." But it was the church that really drilled that lesson home. It was the church—all along the spectrum from fundamentalist to hyper-liberal—that nurtured my voice of constant self-interrogation over whether I was doing "enough."

As a kid at church, I was always hearing that "love is an action, not a feeling," and I think that's true. But within my White upper-middle-class context, I also heard that phrase as a summons to throw the full force of my resources, privilege, and of course my oh-so-important education and well-honed "leadership skills" at other people's problems.

But we cannot love people or a place if we don't care even to *know* our neighbors as whole, interconnected communities and people. Often the action that's actually required is to listen and believe what others tell us about their lives. It is to commit to the *incredibly* slow and steady process of building trust in order to be accountable to others.

If we do not listen deeply and undertake our work with fear and trembling and respect, then we end up founding charities full of privileged people who "help" oppressed people "succeed" by becoming more like them. But love does the opposite: it partners with people in becoming more of *themselves.*

Trying to fix our neighbors is merely replicating imperialism under the guise of charity. But love is the opposite of domination and injustice. To love our neighbor is to trust them when they say what they want and need, to notice and care when systemic forces stand in the way of it, to seek their flourishing as whole people. And to begin to heal the harms of empire is to let joy and justice teach us new definitions of worth and work.

———

Jesus wasn't a fixer.

Presumably, Jesus could have waved a hand over each crowd he encountered and mended all the hearts, spines, bruises, minds, and father-wounds all at once. As a kid, it bothered me that he didn't. How could he witness any amount of suffering and not use his power to change it?

Instead, his work was maddeningly slow. He talked with people and asked them questions. He forgave sins, spit in the mud, posed riddles, and told stories all along the way of his healing journeys. This was the kingdom of God, he said, touching the ragtag rabble, one person at a time.

Jesus wasn't a fixer. He healed people, but not because he was uncomfortable with their pain. He met them face-to-face so they could experience his particular love for them; then he not only healed their bodies but restored them to community. Many of them left behind not only their pain and suffering but also their former status as outcasts. At times the Bible literally says he "gave them back" to their families. Some of them he gave back to themselves.

Jesus was not in the business of making people more productive, tidy, or correct. His healings righted relationships within people through an experience that empowered them to right relationships between themselves and others. I don't believe they were just meant to be object lessons about God's power either. I think Jesus restored honor and dignity to them while they were still sick by seeking them out and declaring them worthy of health and belonging. I think each person Jesus healed was a seed of the kingdom of God.

Jesus didn't wave his magic hands over crowds because it just doesn't work that way. For every obvious disease or injury there's an invisible sufferer, a mental illness, an estranged sibling, and a hundred needs to be known and loved. Mending people on all those dimensions is the work of all those people's lifetimes. Jesus wasn't trying to make everything perfect. Instead, his healing reminded folks of what is possible, while disrupting their ideas of how and through whom—creating the space for more, no less miraculous healings to ripple through their lives.

Jesus knew people were desperate for miracles, but he was constantly asking them to also see his wondrous works as signs of something deeper. He knew all too well from his own life and work that restoring relationships and bringing liberation is not instantaneous or spectacular. Healing is long, hard work. Healing is deeper than fixing. Healing can hurt. But healing is also human.

Empire's drive for efficiency tells us there can, should, and will be a fix for everything. That healing is a waste of time. That we should aspire to go back to normal—to predictable, to productive, to independence.

It's a seductive message, because it's the most natural thing in the world to want to fix. Healing requires us to grieve a past way of being that is lost to us forever. Healing is so, so slow, it can feel like the rest of the world is passing us by. When I fix my washing machine in an hour, I feel accomplished. When I heal an injury over weeks and months, I mostly feel tired and behind. There's nothing wrong with wishing for an easy button. And there's certainly nothing glamorous about uncertainty, un-productivity, or interdependence.

But when we let ourselves be sold the lie that the slow way of healing is defective and unnecessary, or even lazy and selfish, we end up being sold fixes that aren't real. The ways we've devised to make our problems go away and whack everything back to normal are just cover-ups.

We can often keep up that lie to others and even to ourselves for a long time. I know a lot about hiding and ignoring pain. But we can't lie to God, and our bodies keep the score. So many times I've avoided my healing because I thought it would break me—only to later have my half-fixed life come apart at the seams anyway.

Every time we hide from our own healing, we ask others to hide theirs from us. We help perpetuate the false narrative that linear, measurable, picture-perfect successes are normal, and anything else is a failure.

The truth is, things change. That's the way of the universe God made. We think we're supposed to pretend that we can reach some static state of bodily health and relational bliss, but eventually in every part of life we'll experience decay, catastrophe, failure, or lack. And even when we are ultimately able to look back and tell a story of breaking and healing, change still sometimes leaves ugly scars. Being changed ourselves, through the long healing process, is a natural and important and worthy part of life. Healing is twice as hard when we resist or delay it. But when we accept it, we start to find the beauty in becoming healers.

Ultimately, healing is a process we can't skip over, and often one that never ends, but when we accept that, healing also reveals itself as a beautiful, creative, and deeply communal choice. Even with his magic hands, Jesus could only set people down the first steps of the path toward true restoration. He deputizes people he heals as repairers, re-imaginers, reconcilers, re-creators. Today he trusts us, too, to carry out this mission with exactly the tools we're already holding—and with the experience of our worthiness and his love.

When we learn how to cooperate with our own healing processes, we can bring this same wisdom into our relationships, communities, and work. When we are compassionate toward our own pain, we can sit with others in theirs—or even with the world in its groaning—without feeling compelled to fix it for our own comfort. We know that even while the pain is still raging, simply being seen and touched in the midst of it already begins to heal feelings of isolation and shame. We can witness and help to hold pain, and we can hold hope for others when hope seems far out of reach. Those of us who have cried out to God in our loneliest, angriest, and most brokenhearted moments have the power to become people who hold wide open space for others in prayer: space for ragged desperation, for rage, for wild hope, for acceptance and grief, or for all of them at once. Those of us who have made it through, one scrap of solace at a time, have a unique ability to call to the same strength in others when they feel they have none left.

When we begin to learn self-trust toward our bodies, minds, and hearts and their ability to work together to heal us, we can recognize even more places where empire has overlooked and discounted the resources needed to step creatively into the future. With all those hidden resources at our disposal, we start to understand Jesus's stories about people who are bad at math. We're not so scandalized by the landowner who paid the workers of ten-hour, six-hour, and two-hour days all the same wage, because we've glimpsed an economy of grace where "the last will be first, and the first will be last" (Matthew 20:16 NRSV). We can let go of trading an eye for an eye. We become like the shepherd who leaves ninety-nine sheep to find one lost sheep (Matthew 18:12–14), because we recognize the infinite, sacred worth of each person. We experience that "the kingdom of heaven is like yeast that a woman took and mixed into about sixty pounds of flour until it worked all through the dough" (Matthew 13:33)—that the love and justice of God grow from the microscopic to the miraculous.

When we've experienced the depth of slow healing and the strength it brings, we can become voices who value small victories, who choose connectedness, who ask questions and cast visions that look toward sustainable and long-lasting change. We know that sometimes the smallest outward indicator is the first sign of truly radical inward, systemic change. We recognize that a slow and steady process where we remain in integrity—in right relationship and structural soundness—can ultimately have exponentially greater results than an overnight success built on thin relationships and shaky foundations. Just as we come to appreciate the healing power of evenings around a fire with friends, we can call for our churches or political organizations to invest in growing our power and strength through relational and emotional health, interdependence, and joy and play.

For a long time I was told that approaching these communal sins as relational failures gave too much leeway to those who would over-spiritualize them to avoid addressing them concretely. I've shied away from too much talk of "kindness," "awareness," or "compassion" as solutions when those in need would rather have healthcare and an adequate minimum wage.

But to create that kind of change, we need everyone's help. To sustain the effort it would require, we need all kinds of creative gifts, and we need to allow each other to work to sustainable rhythms. We need each other to be inspired and empowered; we need movements where people feel invited and accepted, connected and grounded and cared for. But too often, those vital aspects of political organizing and changemaking don't show up in our strategic plans.

I have also experienced this on the smallest scale: my own spiritual and relational health have turned out to be the strongest predictors of my physical health and overall well-being. Like political organizing, managing a chronic illness is a long, long game with long odds. It may look on the outside as though the right supplements or exercise routine matters most; but outside the context of my prayer practices or my social network of care, those would just be more frustrating items on my to-do list.

Before I tried supporting my body with stress management, food, movement, sleep, and time in community, I assumed that while these things clearly affect human health, pharmaceutical interventions were so much more powerful as to render them irrelevant. That is, after all, how my first doctors went about treating me. But the more side effects I experienced from the drugs, the less I wanted to keep yanking my body's systems around by the most powerful tools available. It felt like sending another Hulk to battle the Hulk. It felt like screaming at an emotionally overloaded person to "CALM DOWN!" It felt like discovering rats in the house, setting loose a horde of snakes, and living with them instead.

It turned out that the gentler supports my body needed *were* just as powerful as the drugs, but they were harder to perceive as such because they worked more slowly and required more of my time, energy, and attention than popping a pill. They also worked *together* over time to help restore my systems' own balance. This process felt only arduous at first but has slowly become a virtuous cycle, not only halting the damage but also healing it and restoring the system to some resilience.

This is a different way of defining "effectiveness" or "efficiency" from the short-term measures we are used to putting on things. But in a world that's become increasingly uncertain, slow and supported change has become the only kind I'm interested in. When it comes to social change, I don't want to be part of burnout-driven "victories" that can be overturned elsewhere the next day. Certain flashpoint moments or superhuman efforts may have their place, but like steroids, their very intensity can also quickly corrode the infrastructure needed to sustain a lasting transformation. When they're most effective, it's because a much broader movement has worked throughout the whole environment to prepare people and systems for a major shift.

Despite what most management consultants would tell us, things like experiencing joy and tending to spiritual needs are not cherries on top of immediate physical interventions; they support and sustain our bodies' systems, our ability to discern what's right, and the rhythms of life that help us continue to prioritize our deepest values. They are the vital foundation of our ability to embody healing.

But, as I learned in some of the hardest months of my life, they're also not things we can do alone.

PART IV

7

COMMUNITY AND OTHER RESCUED BUZZWORDS

When Nate and I moved to Charleston, I shifted to working remotely. We knew no one in town, or even in the state. Soon after my first Behçet's flare, I was laid off from my job, and consequently from my virtual coworking relationships. Now I was sick, friendless, and jobless.

By the end of our first year here, we'd actually made a few friends in town. Then we moved out of our dark, roach-infested apartment, where we'd spent a lot of time with our hallway neighbors. And in another six months, the rest of our friends had all moved away.

With the inevitable resulting feeling of abandonment, my sense of isolation became palpable. I struggled to relax and "be myself" around anyone unfamiliar (i.e., anyone in town), and I felt hyper-focused on my loneliness in my day-to-day life even though I was fully aware it couldn't be "solved" with anything other than time.

Since I was a teenager, I'd been determined to organize my life around deep community. Other people aspire to fame and fortune; I aspire to impromptu neighborly porch beers and long tables surrounded by an unlikely motley crew. As years wore on in Charleston, my loneliness felt like nothing more or less than failure at the most extreme level.

Writing about loneliness feels scary. My brow furrows and my chest tightens when I think about putting my experiences of isolation into words. I once thought they'd be easier to talk about when I finally found myself with a strong support system and a happy, healthy social life. I would say those things are true of me, yet I still feel reluctant both to revisit my years of loneliness and to put them into words that others will read. Maybe I hope those years of sadness and confusion can be witnessed retroactively— but only if I can keep the shame and fear wrapped up in a rag, held close, hidden.

As social mammals, we humans need each other on every level. We depend on each other for food, shelter, and protection—but also for other basic needs, like emotional regulation, or the social connection and relational feedback that help us place our very sense of self. Because we're designed to survive and thrive through cooperation, we experience loneliness as an existential threat.

Loneliness is painful. Our new marriage was happy, beautiful, and #blessed, but I had no one else to process it with. Illness made it that much harder to connect with people. Should I hide this all-consuming reality of my life, or go ahead and drop an awkward bomb at cocktail hour? None of us wants to face this about ourselves, but we shy away from those who are suffering. Meanwhile, I needed help;

I needed to share my weird food with people and not feel weird; I needed interactions with people without the high stakes of a social situation; but I had no one to ask.

Loneliness translates intuitively into shame. Being alone seems to beg the question: What is wrong with you that makes you not belong? And the pain of loneliness is inherently hard to talk about; to confess to loneliness is to make an implicit demand on your confessor. It's something we need other people in order to "solve," and yet it's also something other people can't necessarily solve for us.

I eventually learned that my intense feelings of pain, failure, and shame were actually universal features of the human experience of loneliness. After all, for most of human history, we've lived with small clans, not cities a million strong, so a feeling of such extreme disconnection—signaling loss or exclusion from the safety of the tribe—would have been a sign of a true existential threat. The massive discomfort and fear engendered by loneliness would be a strong motivator to rejoin the group by any means necessary.

In modern times, when we have (seemingly) infinite choice in where we live and whom we associate with, many of the hallmarks of loneliness become maladaptive. The visceral sense of threat we feel translates to social anxiety, and triggers an instinct to self-protect by becoming less trusting and more judgmental of others.

Living in this state is massively stressful to our hearts and minds, but also to our bodies—making loneliness as strong a predictor of disease and death as smoking or sedentariness. Just as importantly, we all know in our own broken hearts how deeply it affects our simple ability to feel connected, to feel like ourselves, to feel alive from day to day.

In the first year or two of learning to manage my illness, drugs, food, and supplements definitely occupied most of my time and attention. Then there was finding a good routine of regular movement within my limits, managing sleep, and coping with stress. But more recently, I've been surprised that I notice real improvement when I also tend to other needs and longings, like feeling connected to others and to nature. In these years of learning how to pay attention to my symptoms, I've found that time with my closest friends and family is a reliable predictor of how I'll feel, particularly how resilient my body will be when faced with other triggers.

Scientists have linked social isolation to increased inflammation, and loneliness to a stronger inflammatory response to stress. Since inflammation leads to autoimmune symptoms, more sources of inflammation will only exacerbate the problem. Inflammation is also a culprit for many other health problems, like heart disease and some cases of depression. On the other hand, human connection is a major ingredient in the body's physical ability to mount a stress response and then return properly to a state of rest and relaxation.

Like "reduce your stress" and "hug more trees," "spend more time with people you love" is one of those pieces of advice that makes a lot of sense and also sounds impossible. Most of the actions people suggest as ways to be more healthy sound simultaneously wishy-washy, self-indulgent, and unachievable. But maybe instead of ignoring this advice, we should ask more questions about what forces in our world are conspiring against our ability to follow it.

————

In the last ten years or so, research on loneliness has grown, and public health officials have started to talk about a "loneliness epidemic" in the United States and beyond. Learning that I was not alone in my loneliness made me feel somewhat less defective and ashamed—but it didn't make me feel less lonely or less sad. Instead, it made my loneliness seem somehow inevitable, a result of forces well beyond my control. While that might relieve some of my anxiety about being an inherently repulsive person, it didn't relieve my nagging, aching sense that this might actually never end.

Since then, I've come to find the "loneliness epidemic" phrase a little tiresome. I love geeking out about public health as much as the next justice-minded chronically ill person, but I struggle with the need to label all our biggest social ills as "epidemics" before they matter. Do we really have a loneliness epidemic, a domestic abuse epidemic, an opioid epidemic, a gun violence epidemic, and on and on, that we can make plans to control and contain like we could if each of these were a discrete microbe? Or do we have a series of interlocking cultural and systemic failures leaving huge segments of our society trapped in chronic pain and ongoing trauma to the point that all these problems overlap and intertwine?

In the case of loneliness, I researched and read about many plans and programs to help bring people together. Some of them seemed well-founded and successful, but even if they existed in my town, none of them would have included me. Besides, I didn't suffer from self-isolation; I "brought myself together" with plenty of people. If there is anything I can say I learned for sure during that time, it's that coffee doesn't solve loneliness. Even the most proactive among us can't one-hour-conversation our way to a strong community and a deep sense of belonging.

Instead, loneliness is a pervasive feature of our culture and our society. It's a problem that inherently requires structural support and widespread awareness in order to change. We can learn how to design for community in our neighborhoods, workplaces, churches, habits, and ways of life. But so many of our structural systems and cultural choices have instead selected for isolation.

Even the neighborhoods we built in the second half of the twentieth century—with bigger and bigger houses, wider streets for cars but fewer sidewalks, and pretty picket fences—cast a vision of prosperity that distanced us from our neighbors. Likewise, the typical early-career trajectory for anyone aspiring to the professional class is expected to include multiple moves from city to city in order to be able to move up the career ladder. We don't hesitate to call it "success" when someone makes it to the C-suite before forty but has never had enough time or stability to belong to a community that cares about them.

We're quick to valorize independence and to devalue or even pathologize interdependence. As Emily and Amelia Nagoski write: "The 'common wisdom' is that individual development should be a linear progression from dependence to autonomy. . . . An identity grounded in autonomy is considered stronger, superior, and masculine. An identity grounded in connection is weaker, inferior, and feminine. . . . [In reality] humans are built to *oscillate* from connection to autonomy and back again." Everyone has the right to provide for their own basic needs without having to put their fate in someone else's hands. At the same time, we all know that ultimately, our fate is always in each other's hands. The pandemic made this clear: without knowing how to cooperate, or to conceive of ourselves as members of a collective, Americans failed to protect each other from COVID-19.

Loneliness is a justice issue: it puts vulnerable people at even further risk. And when marginalized people are kept isolated from each other, they lose not only a source of support but also the ability to organize for political power.

On an even deeper level, we don't just need each other for survival, but also to know who we are. We're accustomed to thinking that the border of our "selves" stops at our skin, but as social animals, we're also composed of the relationships that form us and the communities to which we belong. Have you ever spent time with family or old friends and realized you felt more like yourself than you had in weeks or months? We need those relationships of trust, where we can relax—because we are accepted for who we are, and not excommunicated for our mistakes—to integrate ourselves.

Even physiologically, the mirror neurons in the frontal lobes of our brains are made for "tuning in" to others' physical and emotional states. Failing to be mirrored—to have someone else see and validate our emotions and tend to our needs for safety and connection—can mean the difference between experiencing something as a terrible, painful, life-altering event and experiencing it as a trauma: an insurmountable roadblock to healing and being able to feel alive. But when we have had relationships of trust, where we are mirrored and we learn to mirror others, we are likely to have access to an internal sense of safety and the ability to build more loving relationships throughout our lives.

Still, psychologists can tell us that we belong to each other, but our culture and even our laws remain firmly entrenched in the opinion that human connection and community are optional bonuses, not the stuff of our lives. As a result, we end up tired: building our identities around work because we can't find communities to help us hold them. We end up wasteful: buying stuff we could've borrowed if we just knew our neighbors' names. We end up vulnerable—at the mercy of people who sell the solutions to our problems because we don't have anyone to pool resources and creativity with. And we end up with only a vague sense that there is something more, something not-quite-right about how tired and frustrated we feel. We just keep making and sharing memes about how hard it all is.

———

If I'd been born and gotten sick in Jesus's time, I would be an outcast. My inability to keep up with all the tasks of running a household and my struggle to bear children would have marked me as a shame to my family. Diseases of the skin were especially feared, and I could have been declared ritually unclean. Ours is not the only age to judge people's worth by their productivity, or their belonging by their health.

One day, Jesus was teaching in someone's house when the assembled crowd heard a scraping sound above them—soon, they were flooded with sunlight. Squinting up at the brand-new hole in the roof, they saw the light smothered again and a man-sized bundle being shoved through the hole. They jostled even tighter together as the listeners closest to Jesus scrambled to make way for the paralyzed man on the mat. His friends, determined that he would reach Jesus, had banded together to get him there.

This man was ritually unclean. Uninvited, he didn't belong in someone else's house at all. But his friends were willing to literally break barriers to bring him to the healer. (Somehow, I find myself imagining a pack of nineteen-year-old guys.) They knew this was his chance.

Jesus wasn't offended by all this rule-breaking and property damage; instead, he was moved. Luke says that "when he saw *their* faith, he said, 'Friend, your sins are forgiven'"

(Luke 5:20 NRSV, emphasis mine). Just as he had named an outcast woman "Daughter," now he looked at this man and saw a friend. The man didn't do anything or say anything (except, perhaps, to trust his friends to drop him through a hole!). It was his friends' faith that saved him. It was his identity as a friend that meant he was already whole. By the end of the story, Jesus not only forgives him, but also heals him. His friends' determination, creativity, and care gave him new life.

Jesus didn't only accept social outcasts who crossed dividing lines to where he was; after healing the paralyzed man, he went on to invite himself across a dividing line to another outcast. Where people were excluded in the name of a God who cares more about order than about redemption, Jesus came alongside them in the name of a God of creativity and grace.

Levi was a tax collector on behalf of the occupying empire and its army. He was seen as a traitor to his people, the enforcer of invaders' domination, violence, and theft. He was allowed to enrich himself through dishonest practices— taking from his own people with the blessing of empire. He was wealthy, but he belonged nowhere: looked down on by the Romans, mistrusted and despised by his own Palestinian Jewish people. But Levi wasn't an outcast because of misfortune. He chose this path.

When Jesus first saw him, Levi hadn't even given any indication that he was interested in this wandering teacher. He was sitting at his own tax booth, plying his slimy trade. When Jesus said, "follow me," was it a tender call to Levi's deepest, hidden longings? Or is it just as likely that he simply issued a challenge to a bored and restless businessman? Did he really just say the two words? Did Jesus say this to all the tax collectors he passed?

Something in Jesus spoke to something in Levi, who walked off the job and got in line with the smelly fishermen and Sick Women whom Jesus had also chosen for his entourage.

That evening, Levi had them all over. He shared his ill-gotten wealth with his new friends and old ones. He introduced Jesus to his band of the misfits and the misunderstood—tax collectors "and others," the text says. They were used to censure and opprobrium from the religious establishment; a rowdy bunch, a defiant bunch, cynical except when they were oddly, awkwardly tender.

But the presence of the Teacher attracted scrutiny and whispers all over again. The religious leaders complained to his friends: "How can he claim to lead when he keeps such company?" (One has to wonder if they felt snubbed.)

When I think about these two stories, I would rather see myself as a hapless victim of fate than as a traitorous tax collector. But the truth is, as a White woman, I'm both suspected and guilty of betraying my fellow women in exchange for scraps of privilege from the patriarchy. I have the resources to sequester myself in an enclave of the pragmatic and declare myself misunderstood. And if a rabble-rousing preacher came by, I don't know that I'd go out of my way to see him.

But Jesus could look at the wealthy and see need. He ate with the cynically self-sufficient and detected their hidden sickness. And so he cut in on the whisperers and gossips: "It is not the healthy who need a doctor, but the sick. I have not come to call the righteous, but sinners" (Mark 2:17).

It's a more flattering answer than some of his rejoinders to religious leaders. They can walk away thinking themselves "healthy" and "righteous," if they want. I can imagine Jesus throwing the remark over his shoulder, too busy enjoying Levi's hospitality to bother with the nosy and the self-righteous.

Was it the unbotheredness they couldn't stand? Did they seize upon the doctor comment, insisting that real medicine has to be painful and mortifying? They weren't satisfied: "Even your loony cousin's buddies have the decency to fast and pray. What is all this partying about?"

Jesus is still patient. "We are celebrating," he says. "Something new is taking place. We grieve when it is time to grieve, and we party when it's time to party!" (see vv. 18–20).

I think between the lines, he is also saying: *No one was ever shamed and excluded into the loving, just ways of God's kingdom. And we have just as much to learn from our joy and desire as we do from our pain. And what does it feel like for us not to need your permission? And do you know you are invited too?*

Jesus was not just a man of sorrow but also of celebration. He was not just temperate but also excessively joyful. He was at home not just among the meek and mild but also with the raucous and even the rapacious. He could be all of those things. We can be all of those things.

———

After we moved to Charleston, I got sick, we made new friends, and the friends moved away. I slowly slid into a depression and then suddenly had a bit of a breakdown. By the end of our second year here, my loneliness had come to occupy more and more of my mental real estate and began to seem more and more inescapable. I went on a long road trip to see friends and family members. I quit my part-time church job and started a small group. I went to therapy.

A few months later, I sat across a table from my friend Katie and tried to articulate what I'd been noticing about my loneliness and my body since then: a low, humming social anxiety, a hyper-alert and wary feeling I could easily mask to *function* in social situations but often couldn't move beyond to actually *connect* with people. I'd continued to make new friends, but I always felt like I was interacting with them from slightly outside myself, at a tiny remove:

"It's like this tightness in my chest, like this barrier in my mind; I think my body is maybe trying to protect me? Like after so many years of moving around, after all this *leaving*, I've finally blown the fuse on my capacity for loving people and letting them go."

Katie lives with chronic illness and a history of trauma, and she asks the most wonderful questions from the kindest heart. I felt so relieved to even be able to describe what I felt to someone who—if she hadn't felt exactly the same things—would still be able and willing to empathize. Even as we talked about books and theology, I practiced exhaling deeply and relaxing the muscles of my face, embodying openness and curiosity toward my friend just as she demonstrated it to me. "We still have the capacity for love and risk," I silently told my body and my heart. "We are safe here."

It was January 15, 2020.

8

HEALING IS SHARED

Since the pandemic began, the entire concept of loneliness has taken on depths and dimensions most of us could hardly fathom before. Many of us feel the weight, not only of physical isolation, but societal abandonment, as basic protections, assistance, and agreements about how to live together disappear. Parents of young children, essential workers, disabled and immunocompromised people, multi-generational households, and so many more feel totally forgotten. Even if the pandemic ended, we'd be haunted by the truth that so many policymakers—and so many of our neighbors—were more than willing to leave us behind in order to pretend that things were okay.

Nate and I were lucky to have already had a small neighborhood-based church group that met for dinner every Friday night. The crowded table shifted to a big circle in the backyard. As time wore on, there was often little we could do, materially, to help each other. Sometimes, exhausted, we spent much of the evening in silence—together, six feet apart. For that week or that day or that hour, though, it was enough.

Few things have made me feel like I was peering past the end of the world like this did: making a fire and setting out all the blankets we owned so we could still see our friends when it was thirty degrees out. But just like the fire, like a mask or a pill, this is part of how we've survived: by gathering, asking and listening, to remind each other there is yet more in life than bleary eyes, heavy headlines, and the fearsome echo of our own lonely hearts.

After years of this, resources feel so depleted it seems that maintaining any kind of community—let alone striving for any particular quality of community—would be nothing short of a miraculous gift. Yet a few of my friendships *have* grown and flourished, despite the difficulties of distancing, particularly with some sick and disabled friends. While it's nice to be able to share some of the common elements of our experiences, that actually may not be the reason I find their friendship so life-giving. What feels just as present in our relationships is a different perspective on friendship, work, and the world. They are people who know the value of a morning chat on the porch, even when we feel too busy; who are teaching me how to ask for help; who recognized a long game of survival sooner than the rest of us did.

In a long game of survival, your community isn't just the cherry on top of a nice life, or the thing that falls away when you focus on your family. They become your childcare, rideshare, and your garden-bartering network. They're the safety net that allows you to take a medical leave or quit an abusive job. Shared laughter and tears become your mental health support and your fuel for another day.

I'm now lucky to have plenty of friends I could potentially ask for help with something, but I can *always* turn to my chronically ill friends with a need and know we share a life that is necessarily interdependent with others'. Even if it's just a need for prayer, I trust my friends who've lived with deep and abiding pain to know what it's like to not be able to lift ourselves up.

My chronically ill friends are the people in my life who know how to stay. When it's easier to bring a casserole once than to walk beside someone in pain for years, when self-help gurus counsel their disciples that "successful people spend their time with successful people," when we and our bodies remain inconvenient, they stay. They are the ones with time in their lives for friendship. They're the ones I can talk to about my fears of getting sicker and my fears of becoming a hypochondriac. In a world that idolizes choice and change, we are the ones who have the willingness and the practice to keep choosing what we've already chosen: each other.

Our community also has a different relationship to work, achievement, time, and healing. We don't always go from victory to victory, as others feel pressured to (appear to) do. We live in in-betweens, in cycles, in back-and-forths with our physical—and often our mental—health. So we're a little more used to work and relationships that happen on fluid timelines and in shifting patterns too. We learn together how to schedule and reschedule our meetups around illness cycles and flares, or how to gently check in on each other when we've fallen off the grid into a bout of pain or depression.

When I'm with my able-bodied friends, I think often of the many times during my lonely years that I filled up my days with work, volunteering, and activities just to distract myself from my loneliness. I wanted to actively resist a culture of isolation. Not knowing how, I eventually willingly succumbed to it, intentionally chasing "success" because I had failed to find what I really wanted: community. When we're able to, we *default* to a life that centers on pursuing an individual career, and tries to fit everything else in around that.

My chronically ill friends know what it is like to *not be able* to always pursue a bigger, better career or more Instagrammable consumerism, and to *have to* make meaning out of a life oriented around something else. Like so many other groups of people who don't fit into "normal," we're always making our own rhythms, patterns, and unspoken understandings. In these small pockets, we can create space together that works for us—our own, more inclusive normal.

Having a place where we are allowed, accepted, and accommodated is fun, pleasurable, and meaningful, but it is also immensely *empowering*. This is true on an individual level—interdependence increases the resources available to each of us—but it is also a collective reality. The most sustainable and effective activist movements I've been a part of recognized that belonging, safety, care, kindness, and joy— practices for what Martin Luther King Jr. and his mentor Howard Thurman named "Beloved Community"—are our most important resources and tools in our long, difficult fights for justice.

Without community and creativity, activists for justice are merely playing by the rules of a game that's rigged against us. That game defines power as having lots of resources and influence with the "right" people. Too often, we define "effectiveness" as chasing after those things in order to pass our next legislation or sway public opinion. But when we're organizing with poor folks or on behalf of the land, we're always facing opposition from corporations and anyone who benefits from keeping things the way they already are. We can never out-resource corporate lobbyists and career politicians. We must draw on another source of power.

Some of us are quick to *say* that our true power lies in our vision for a more humane way of living, in the fact that the great majority of us long for true peace and right relationship. We might say we build power through song, through mutual aid and care, through art and unlikely friendships— through community that multiplies into more than the sum of its parts. But when it comes to the daily work of growing and deploying power to make change, we don't always act like we believe these things. We can get so caught up in our short-term, measurable, external goals, we never quite get around to cultivating the qualities of Beloved Community within our movements. When we feel like we're "winning," we say we must keep the momentum going. When we think we're "losing," we double down.

We do the same in our churches when we prioritize church growth and programming over prayer, care, and the spiritual growth and community-building that happens outside formal channels. Even a version of "discipleship" that looks like "becoming your Best Self" becomes a distraction from imperfectly following the Holy Spirit in our real lives ever farther into grace. We talk about community but never really dare each other to ask for help. We preach about rest then hustle the board into meeting on a Sunday again.

Then, when our leaders and colleagues burn out on this incessant doing, we ask them to politely take some time off and come back when they're ready. Burnout is an endemic problem in churches, nonprofit spaces, and movements for justice, which we routinely insist on treating as an individual issue. We admonish each other about "self-care" and pretend that is the same as caring.

More and more of us are saying, *we can't go on this way.* And we are learning to point to the roots of these issues in ableism and White supremacy, tied up with toxic colonial capitalism—the mindset of extraction. Still, we are sometimes so constrained by those very cultures and systems, we don't quite know how to imagine a different way of being together and doing our work.

———

Jesus gathered an unlikely crew. The fishermen, the wealthy women, the Zealot—an armed political radical whom empire would have labeled a "terrorist." The tax collectors, the Romans, and the pansy-ass Pharisees who met with him by night. These people should not have gotten along; by all accounts of the early church, they didn't. But Jesus insisted that they love one another.

Somehow, he believed this deeply weird little community was more than the sum of its parts. If he were a cleverer religion-founder, he would've capitalized on his fame with a dramatic final address to the adoring crowds that followed him everywhere. Instead, he gave his farewell speech to his twelve ride-or-dies, in the form of a foot-washing. He told them to take care of each other, with an urgency behind his eyes. He seemed to feel that if they could just do that— despite the violence, judgment, and temptation that surrounded them—his mission would be complete. There in the end, he made no distinction between that mission and his simple, deep, iron-forged love for his friends. He trusted that there was real power in what they had.

In the White, Western church of my experience, we seem to have good intentions, or at least hopes, of forming this kind of mismatched, grace-filled community; but we struggle to find and foster it. Historically, that's because we've failed to attend to power. As the privileged sect of the modern empire, we've lost our sensitivity to hidden power imbalances and our intuition for the wisdom that comes from the special vantage point of the margins. We claim to want "multiethnic" churches when really we want a comfortable minority of minorities in an organization led by White values. We say we are going to befriend the poor, but we never get beyond "serving," pitying, and trying to help them be more like us.

But Jesus, the healer, felt no compunction to fix anyone. He took the position of humility by receiving Levi's lavish hospitality. He wasn't so afraid someone at the party might do a sin that he couldn't just enjoy an evening together. More than he had some grand rescue plan for Levi or even a point to make to anyone, I think Jesus just liked to eat, drink, and cut up. More than he wanted Levi to experience the expansive feeling of "being a good person," he helped Levi experience the never-ending celebration of the kingdom of God, the simple grace of acceptance and respect.

Some of us who've learned more about the insidious workings of power and privilege have not yet caught on to ways of practicing something else. Without another frame of reference, we have capitulated to empire's lie that the opposite of unearned power and privilege is self-silencing, worthlessness, and subjection. Having gotten it wrong before, we're too ashamed to try again. Having belatedly recognized our ill-gotten gains, we still fail to humbly accept the gifts of God. We convince ourselves we're too tainted to belong at the feast of the motley gang. Having spent so long believing ourselves to be righteous, we're still somehow afraid we might do a sin.

When I became the man on the mat, I had to reckon with the ways I was still letting power and privilege define me even as I'd thought I was trying to resist them. Instead of chasing after money and success in my early twenties, I'd farcically hustled for my worth in what I thought was the opposite direction. But in fact, the opposite of hustle is stillness. The opposite of unearned privilege is simple human need. The opposite of the world's version of power isn't weakness; it's the power of vulnerability and of the connection that results. The opposite of grounding my identity in Whiteness and middle-class success isn't grounding my identity in resisting those things; it's grounding my identity in the love and acceptance of Jesus. That is where true humility can put down roots, making way for connection and community to blossom.

———

Our bodies draw us into communion with the world. Our five senses are the only ways we have to connect with others, and so often it is our bodies' labor, creativity, mealtimes, or physical environments that introduce us to those who become our dearest friends. And, of course, the families into which we are born are stories of our ties to other bodies.

Science, observation, and sense have shown me that my own body flourishes best in proximity to those of my born and chosen kin. But really, we all know this about ourselves. We've all known skin hunger—and the healing power of touch. We all have longed for someone with a visceral ache. We've barely realized we were white-knuckling our way through a day or week, until a moment with a friend helped us breathe again.

That's why it's so tragic that our society has also made bodies into sites of exclusion, injustice, othering, and oppression. Those with Black, Brown, Indigenous, and other bodies of color, queer and trans bodies, disabled bodies, women's bodies, fat bodies, and more must often find ways to welcome and embrace *ourselves* and each other precisely because the wider world has marked our bodies as different, exploitable, or expendable. Yet even as we unlearn these stories about ourselves, we're also reminded that our bodies tell the sacred stories of who we are, draw us together with those who have common embodied experiences, and continue to bear us through our lives with the inviolable dignity of the very image of God. It is often in reclaiming these truths *together* with similarly othered people and their bodies that we find some of our most tender, truest, holiest healing and joy. In this way, so many minoritized groups have found their own ways to survive and thrive outside of mainstream, colonial visions of "success." Those of us who've been pushed outside the "normal" ways of living have already experimented, tried, failed, and surprised ourselves, all on faith, because that was all we had.

I've found that it's easy for Christians to accidentally "community shame" each other. I often hear friends sigh and say, "I should invite more of my neighbors over," or "I just haven't had time to volunteer like I should." While community does require consistency and sometimes discipline, it's also not served by blaming or shaming ourselves about a structural problem. It seems like we all want to know the four action steps guaranteed to sweep us into authentic community; but we also dread trying to tack them onto our to-do lists when our real quest is for something so much deeper.

I think in our hearts we know that community is not a goal we reach simply by adding more people to our calendars; it's a way of life. When we follow the lead of marginalized people who already live it, we discover that we can share an abundance of creative and caring ways forward.

When my first friends moved away, I got invited to another dinner group, a table of Black women and White women of all ages who'd gotten together for honest conversations about race. Against all the odds, we've gone from a gathering for "race conversations" to simply a group of dear friends who aren't afraid to talk about how race and racism affect our daily lives.

We've learned that community ultimately forms out of two ingredients: time and trust. In some ways, community is the most practical, action-oriented thing in the world; but there are no shortcuts, especially if we hope to form deep connection across difference. Wherever we have to beg, borrow, or steal the time, relationships must be nurtured in consistency. And however many times we have to show up to the hard conversation or small act of care, there is no substitute for hard-earned trust.

We also earn trust and deepen relationship by attending to access. Friendship, community, and mutual aid aren't magic solutions to injustice—but especially not when contexts of power and privilege can't be acknowledged or their patterns interrupted. When we are entrusted with friendship with someone who experiences a form of oppression we don't, people of privilege have the joy of listening, practicing humility, and offering to walk alongside in advocacy.

In community with my sick and disabled friends, I've learned to notice the accessibility of spaces I enter. In their company, growing radical compassion for my own body has helped me meet others' bodies with care, respect, and wonder; being in loving community with others' bodies has grown my patience and love for my own. And while these practices and experiences are beautiful among friends, they're also incomplete unless we're extending those values into our churches, workplaces, and other spaces by making sure *everyone* has what they need to participate joyfully.

In my own impatient, abled past, I might have sympathized with the person or organization that treats accessibility needs as massive impositions. But now that I have more disabled, fat, elderly, and mentally and physically ill friends than ever before, I've learned how vanishingly few of those needs are actually difficult to remember, understand, or implement. It's an honor to be with each other and an honor to be able to care for each other by accommodating each other's bodies and needs. Accommodations don't just benefit individuals. They set a tone of welcome for an entire space, saying: Bodies are seen and honored here. Differences are celebrated here. All of you belongs here.

When we're oblivious or unresponsive to people's accommodation needs, we send the opposite message: We unwittingly enforce conformity and exclude valuable voices—sacred human beings. We're asking people to check parts of themselves at the door and enter if they dare.

Changing that is as simple as asking a few questions and implementing a few habits at a time. Is there seating in your house that's comfortable for fat bodies? Can you include allergen labels and/or a few varied choices in your snack spread? Can you add image descriptions and video captions to your social media posts? Will you raise some questions about accessibility at your workplace?

Committing to accessibility requires us to let go of myths: that "effectiveness" always means "the quickest path to victory over our opponents"; that exhibiting care for our friends and neighbors is less "radical" or political than advocating for large groups or for strangers; that rest, comfort, dignity, and access are too frivolous to pursue until the "real work" is done; that some roles count for more than other, expendable or low-status roles; that burnout is normal, and it is normal for nearly everyone to struggle to access long-term sustainability in our work together.

These myths obscure the truths that the soonest, most effective change we will ever make is within ourselves and with our families and friends. Whenever we care for each other, we are embodying our dreams for the world. This work is just as "real" as any legislative victory or media campaign. Every role in the wide ecosystem of our movements should be dignified and honored, and we need leaders who can model moving among them, stepping forward and stepping back with grace rather than clamoring for status.

To fully embrace this way of life, we have to let go of old ideas about what growth and change should look like. We might have to redefine efficiency to reprioritize integration and integrity instead of speed alone. We might have to loosen our grip on strict definitions of what is "evidence-based" in order to also include the knowledge of ancestors, of communal wisdom, of bodies and intuitions. We might have to unlearn the metaphor of "progress" itself until it is able to embrace the nonlinear and the cyclical, the slow and steady, deep and invisible, the smallest-scale shift and the seventh generation of change.

Accessibility can be painstaking work that mirrors the seemingly slow and fiddly daily practice of self-compassion and other-love; but it is this kind of fidelity to our values and to one another that grows our collective integrity. This deep-rootedness and right relationship allow us to grow things that both last and adapt—the keys to remaining for the long haul.

As these slowly become second nature, we are being formed in the way of hospitality, solidarity, and care. We grow our sensitivity to the presence and organization of bodies in every space we enter. And we cultivate the discipline of treating every body as sacred and every person as worthy and welcome.

After all, we are all only temporarily abled. Illness, injury, and age come for everyone. What would it feel like to help create a world where—among all the things we might fear about the breakdown of our bodies—exclusion and isolation didn't have to be one of them?

I think it would feel like belonging. Like dignity. Like peace. Like a more resilient sort of Wholeness.

PART V

9

EARTH AND OTHER PRICELESS TRASH HEAPS

In 2017 I watched Hurricane Irma churn across the Atlantic Ocean toward my home in Charleston, South Carolina, as autoimmune flares ravaged my body. The widening gyre on the screen felt familiar, somehow: a weather system, not only caught in a naturally occurring feedback loop, but in one exacerbated by climate change. As the hurricane rolled across my laptop screen, I knew her—I recognized her—I was her. Her ferocity, her uncontrollable rage lived inside me, in my disease. In my body, who saw her, who knew her grief, who knew her inexorability.

I felt dread but also respect for this spiral of tropical rage, at that time the most powerful hurricane ever recorded. After we evacuated from our home, Irma changed course and missed us. But other hurricanes have increasingly been pushed farther north by changing ocean currents, putting

South Carolina more directly in a line of fire that used to extend along the southern coast of Florida.

I escaped Irma. But I could not escape my body. I knew that Irma would resurrect herself over and over, that this was a cycle, that it did not end—that the heat and light and toxic waste and indifference that had created her would go on, and it would rise again and again in spirals of rage.

In the same way, I knew the destruction that lived inside of me and its demand for a witness would not be put off; it might relent, but it would not end. I not only had to know it, recognize it, appease it, or accept it, but somehow, also, in some way, in the way that I feared it—also to love it. A hurricane is not an aberration of the hot, pulsing ocean; neither is my disease an aberration of my wise and angry body.

No one intended to send my body's systems spiraling out of control, any more than they intended to catastrophically alter the earth's climate. Still, I felt in my bones that flash of recognition at the ocean's desperate rage; my immune system, too, was unleashing its own awe-ful force upon my life. We'll never know for certain all the precise causes of Hurricane Irma or my Behçet's disease; but we do know environmental degradation by humans is a major factor in the background of both. Just like hurricanes are a natural, seasonal phenomenon that's occurring more frequently with more strength due to climate change, evidence that autoimmune disease is on a sharp rise points to environmental factors causing autoimmune-inducing genes to express ("switch on") more often—especially in the developed world.

After the hurricane, I found in every swelling joint, in every open pustule of skin, grief—the grief of the world. I felt the rage of the ocean washing through my own inflamed blood vessels. And I vowed to honor it all.

Perhaps I did this, at first, still with the sense that it could end; that something about these spirals of destruction could be laid neatly to rest, with enough attention, enough belief, enough giving and letting go; and I set out to do it all. And while it was, indeed, enough, to lend some peace, some healing, some lessening of the uncontrollable destruction, it would never quite make things go back to the way they were. I learned that nothing will ever go back to the way it was.

Yet I also learned to hold the splintered, shattered bits of things destroyed and find that there was still holiness within them; there was still grace to be met within this storm and truth to be told from inside of disease.

————

When we evacuated for Hurricane Irma, the earth was on my mind. I'd been knee-deep in navigating the Autoimmune Protocol, an elimination diet that has shown success in clinical trials in treating some autoimmune diseases by identifying foods that might contribute to inflammation. In paying close attention to every bite that went into my mouth, I was newly hyper-aware that every cell of my body was made of soil and sun.

By the time I got sick, I was inching our family toward vegetarianism, learning to make sourdough, and in a local community-supported farm share. Ethics were part of it, but this way of eating also made me happy. And it all fell apart when I suddenly reduced my diet to meat and bone broth, coconuts, and non-nightshade vegetables. In all my years of carefully considering where my food came from, I had barely even considered the whole nutrition side of food shopping. I'd even been a little creeped out by the obsessions with "clean" eating and "pure" foods, as if everything (and everyone) else in the store could be somehow tainted. Now I was (and remain today) the lady in the aisle sifting through ingredients lists for allergens and oils, preservatives and thickeners, organic and gluten-free labels or lack thereof.

The elimination diet was a way of performing a scientific experiment on myself to determine what foods might cause an inflammatory response—a process I'm still in, years later. But I also wanted to know why certain foods might trigger autoimmune reactions, and why others might help protect against them. Nutrition science is still in its infancy, and our understanding of the gut microbiome is much, much younger; but some of the theories I read about back at the beginning of this journey seem to have played out in my own life.

First, eliminating foods is only half of the Autoimmune Protocol; it's also meant to focus on adding more nutrient-dense foods to your life. I wasn't only downing weird stuff like bone broth because I needed the calories, but also because animal bones contain so many vital nutrients that we normally just throw away. In fact, I also ate beef liver or other organ meats once a week for the same reason. If my digestive system was out of whack, part of the process of healing would not only be eliminating foods that screwed it up but also adding tons of nutrients to replace those my body was missing when it was failing to digest food well.

The other half of AIP was removing gluten, grains, legumes, sugar, alcohol, dairy, soy, nightshade vegetables, nuts, seeds, and seed spices from my diet. As someone who'd been trying to edge my way toward vegetarianism for the sake of the planet, eliminating grains and legumes was a massive shift.

Drinking the liquefied bones of animals somehow felt more viscerally predatory than eating a chicken breast. But

I also found it fascinating and comforting, being compelled to cook and eat offal, confronting and reversing the food waste involved in my usual, standard American approach to eating meat. I'd always theoretically liked the idea of trying to make use of a whole animal, both from the planetary-conservation standpoint of reducing waste and also from the perspective that it is a way to honor the animal. There's a massive gulf between the practice of grabbing a factory-farmed, factory-rendered, neatly displayed steak from the store shelf without a second thought, and appreciating a cow's body and life enough to make sure it continues to contribute to the web of life as much as possible. But apart from a few brave farmer's market forays, I'd never quite gotten around to learning to cook and eat the weirder cuts of meat.

For the same reason—nutrient density—I went in search of local, pasture-raised meat. Not only was it easier to buy offal from a local supplier; animals who munch grass or forage for insects all day also consume and contain more nutrients than those who are trapped in barns and fed corn-based feed.

As someone who cares about ethics, I'm embarrassed to say I'd previously never gotten around to finding a source of meat from animals who lived happy lives and died low-stress deaths. I theoretically found factory farming abhorrent, and I had hypothetical goals to pay a premium for meat produced in a better way. But it was inconvenient and expensive, with mostly only the intangible "benefit" of feeling better about myself.

I probably even believed, theoretically, that my physical health depended on the health of the land, plants, and animals from which I ate. But only when I got sick did I experience that truth in my own marrow. I had managed a food pantry, worked in catering, and studied food and environmental systems at the graduate level, but I'd never deeply entered into my own relationship with my food.

One of my earliest experiences in understanding food systems' interconnected structures, behaviors, and outcomes was my experience of living on a poverty wage and using SNAP (food stamps) while working at a food pantry in Syracuse, New York. To stock our shelves every week, the pantry received a delivery or went to pick up our order from the regional food bank warehouse. As I asked more questions and got more involved in the process, I learned that we could buy food at extremely cheap prices, not only because we bought it in bulk from another nonprofit, but primarily because most of the food was technically waste. We offered vegetables the USDA had bought and canned as a subsidy to keep them off the market and prop up prices, and cereals that had been overproduced and were now in someone's way (but became a tax write-off if donated). We bought grab bags of frozen meat by the pound, and logged on to our weekly ordering site extra-early to get dibs on quickly ripening produce that local farmers couldn't get to market in time.

I loved spending time with our regulars and volunteers, and our operation met an immediate need for hungry people. But over the course of the year I went from feeling that we were a positive force in the world to viewing our shelves with frustration and sadness. In its full context, our work helped people, but only by giving them what they should have been able to afford for themselves in the first place—and only through a time-consuming and even humiliating process. We were a stopgap patch on a system that deliberately wastes food and calls it charity; a conscience soother for a country that perpetually threatens to cut food stamps, but then has to spend the same amount to fund food banks and pantries struggling to alleviate the hunger that results. We were burdened with screening people to keep them from "taking advantage of the system," as if crowds were clamoring to come sit in our church basement between the hours of 9 and 11 on Friday mornings, waiting to choose between canned green beans and canned carrots.

When I'm driving all over town for expensive groceries, I often think about the food pantry and my own SNAP card from those days. I think about the time and energy it took to feed myself at all, the judgment and disdain I faced for being on welfare, the way I'd plan a whole week's budget around a single container of local yogurt from the farmer's market. It wouldn't have mattered whether I believed that "food is medicine" or whether I wanted to increase the nutrient density of my diet when my access to food was strictly limited to the cheapest options available.

Today, having to pay attention to the ingredients and provenance of every bite—but more importantly, having to pay attention to my body's responses—has changed the way I experience conversations about food systems. My "relationship with food" went from the theoretical realm to the immediate, the bodily, the sub-verbal depths of my literal gut. In fact, while elimination diets are not for everyone, mine became a gateway into what I'd later learn to name as "intuitive eating." Through the reintroduction process, I slowly learned to notice what makes my body feel good (and what doesn't) and honor what she craves, rather than trying to make her conform to someone else's food rules. Once again, she showed me she could be trusted.

These practices, of attunement with my body and choosing food grown in right relationship with land and animals, began to grow my sense of my own creatureliness. It is humbling, in a way, and immensely freeing, to recognize that your body belongs to nature. I may want to be an extra-righteous vegetarian, but my body is an omnivore. And yet, not just an omnivore—she belongs to a whole food web, so that the literal health of the soil, the grass, the insects, and the chicken directly affect hers. Her desires don't merely map onto a set of inputs and outputs, or even a moment-to-moment series of cravings and sensations; they are one of millions of factors working together in our ecosystem, this ecosystem, the Lowcountry. My body lives well when the land lives well.

When we think in systems, we have to be willing to engage with small-scale solutions while also keeping an eye on the big picture. Whether or not we feel particularly beholden to the microbes under the soil, or alarmed by factory farming's contributions to climate change, environmental justice is more than a spiritual project; it is also essential to many of our urgent issues of human rights. If nourishing food is so essential to human life and health, then it is a human right. But increasing access to good food will ultimately involve big investments in changes that will affect the entire global food system.

As with every system outlined in this book, today's poor—in the United States and developing countries—bear the brunt of environmental devastation and food injustice. I may consider myself spiritually "disconnected" from my food, but subsistence farmers in India are literally losing their land to US chemical corporations, while the 2.4 million people experiencing food apartheid in the United States have minimal access to a grocery store that offers fresh food and produce.

Environmental health directly affects public health. Problems like climate change and deforestation cause disasters that most directly affect some of the poorest people in the world. Hunger and malnutrition stemming from poverty and food apartheid hurt children's academic and social development. Access to green space in urban areas can mean better air quality and better mental health. In every place where we nurture the land, we improve the quality of life for humans, because we belong to the land. We are earth.

For centuries, theologians and scientists have warned that when we believe we have comprehension and control over the natural world, our hubris will become our downfall. All the tiny ripples we can't measure and all the downstream effects we don't anticipate accumulate somewhere. And one place, I've learned, is my body.

Some would say I'm just collateral damage. But I believe I'm a canary in a coal mine—more sensitive to dangers that affect all of us in ways we don't entirely understand. Developed countries suffer from rising rates of autoimmunity, but also of other chronic illnesses, infertility, allergies and intolerances, and mental illness. Theories abound as to why: parabens, plastics, and antibacterial soap are to blame; it's something in the water, it's something in the food, it's something in the building materials.

Likely, many of these theories are right and many are wrong. But taking all the raw evidence of disease prevalence together, it's hard to avoid the conclusion that something about our lives in these countries deemed "successful" is slowly eating many of us alive from the inside. In our society's quest to fill those shelves with such a huge variety of food and sell it at a profit, food has become a consumer good rather than a sacred gift of the earth. Farming has become a cost-cutting business rather than a vocation to care for the land. Eating has become a chore done in isolation rather than a communal experience. And anything more has become a luxury rather than an essential part of a whole human life.

We all entrust our health to farmers, honeybees, store stockists, and the water cycle. Each of our bodies belongs to a specific ecosystem, even as we also participate in the great biosphere of planet Earth. These bodies connect us in the most literal sense to hundreds and thousands of other lives. Other systems at whose intersections we live can come to feel amorphous and ephemeral, but the food system—and by extension, the entire ecosystem—indisputably affects our bodies three times a day. We are made of the stuff of other lives.

———

Our ecosystem-existence wove itself even more into the fabric of my life as I realized, over and over, that learning to feed myself well meant learning to feed my 300 trillion bacteria well. Human digestion not only tolerates, but depends upon, these colonies of microbiota. Friendly bacteria help break down food, and they also form part of the mucous lining of the intestines that acts as a barrier between undigested particles and the rest of the body. While our understanding of the gut microbiome is still extremely limited, more and more evidence points to connections between gut dysbiosis—an imbalance of friendly bacteria vs. invaders—and autoimmune disease. As the place where most foreign material enters the body, the digestive tract hosts the majority of immune cells in the human body. Problems with the complex digestive system, its bacterial helpers, or the barriers separating it (and the toxins it filters) from the rest of the body can all cascade into problems for the immune system. For example, one function of friendly bacteria is simply to crowd out invaders, but if their population falters, opportunistic bacteria can get a foothold, further upset the system's balance, and spread into the rest of the body, causing autoimmune reactions. Or if the gut lining is in disrepair, particles can escape the digestive system into the rest of the body, where the immune system interprets them as invaders and attacks.

Gut bacteria even influence mental health—once again, a discovery new enough that a connection has been established even though all of its exact details and mechanisms remain unclear. Patients with depression and anxiety, for instance, are likely to harbor a different gut microbial profile than those without. These disorders are associated with inflammation (a baseline feature of autoimmunity). They could also be affected by gut health via hormones and neurotransmitters produced in the digestive tract, or via the vagus nerve, a part of the emotional brain that extends into the digestive system and connects it with the rest of the brain.

These discoveries disrupt ways of thinking about ourselves that divide our being neatly into parts, especially when those parts are placed in implicit hierarchies. Our rational brains don't simply rule over our emotional centers and our bodies. Instead, we have learned that we are infinitely interrelated within ourselves—and that other beings (microflora) literally constitute part of ourselves—demolishing neat distinctions between mental, physical, spiritual, and relational health.

As scientists attempt to unravel these interrelations and hope for more precise treatment options, we already know some basic principles for supporting gut health: reducing potentially inflammatory or disruptive foods and increasing nutrient density, along with possibly using specialized, targeted antibiotics to kill bad bacteria and supplementing with good ones (probiotics). Both human cells and bacteria in the gut have short lifespans, so continually "feeding" the friendly bacteria that are already present is one of the most important pieces of this puzzle. As humans have coevolved with our favorite symbiotic bacteria, the same nutrient-dense diets that can fortify us also encourage a balanced inner ecosystem.

———

When I was first learning about all these barely understood, intricate moving parts, I felt massively overwhelmed. What was anyone supposed to actually do with all this information? How would I ever know if I'd achieved the "right" microbial profile? How pasture-raised is pasture-raised enough? Does an episode of depression or anxiety signal that I've failed?

At the same time, embarking (skeptically) on this journey at this particular moment in history—when we know just enough to know what we don't know—has also provided the opportunity to continue paying attention to my body rather than pinning all my hopes on someone else's rules and predictions for how my body "should" behave. As years wear on, I've come to realize my healing depends not on getting mired in all the details all the time, but on supporting and being supported by all the systems—from body-mind systems to food systems—to which I belong. Maybe someday someone will be able to tell me exactly which probiotics to take, and whether carrots or blueberries offer the precise nutrient profile my body needs most—but the more I learn about all these interrelated processes, the less likely it seems. Instead, I see how all this complexity creates resilience (either carrots or blueberries are perfectly good) and offers just as much opportunity for positive feedback loops in the direction of healing as that of suffering. Feeding my body mindfully can help with physical symptoms and lead to better mental health, helping me continue to make kind food choices while my body comes to crave carrots and strawberries . . . These choices aren't about calibrating everything to fix my body but about nurturing reciprocal relationships with all the ecosystems in which my body is just one part.

This perspective invites us, once again, not to think about health as an individual pursuit or purchase, but as a project that's inherently relational. Ultimately, whatever food rules I initially followed were only scaffolding that helped me learn new ways of "knowing" about and experiencing my food, my body, and the relationships between them. My experiences and my research taught me that there's no such thing as a goal of a "nutrient dense diet" without any concern for the many beings involved in producing that diet, and even for the ecosystems that surround them. "Going gluten-free" isn't a fad diet for me; it's become a practice of remembering that my health is directly tied to that of the land, animals, and people around me—and around the world.

————

Jesus knew the land that produced his food. He wove parables about soil, foraged for food along dusty roads, and told his followers to be mindful of the seasons, the lilies, and the sparrows. Like most people in ancient times, he was familiar

with the rhythms of the agricultural year and the requirements of a successful garden. As a wandering preacher traveling on foot, he was intimate with the land.

Israel had always had laws about living lightly on the
land. Farmers were required to leave land fallow one year
of every seven to care for its long-term health, and animals
were as entitled to a weekly Sabbath as humans. Religious
festivals followed the agricultural year. Even armies had
to operate within limits to respect relationship with land:
Deuteronomy 20:19 commands them not to cut down fruit
trees when building siege works against an enemy city.

The ancient Jewish people saw creation as God's work of
art, one that was fully alive and offered its own worship to
the Creator, with psalms that depict land and animals, crops
and heavenly bodies all praising God in their own ways. The
nation came to see their land and its flourishing as central to
their identity; and when they envisioned the coming reign
of God's Wholeness, they envisioned a peaceful and pros-
perous place of mutual relationship, with flowing waters,
flourishing trees, plentiful harvests—and secure and joyous
people, the land's caretakers.

In Jesus's time, though, Israel's land—like so much land
belonging rightfully to Indigenous people in the United
States and around the world today—was under occupation
by empire. The people and their place were ruled by faraway centers of power, under the control of soldiers who
had no connection to the land or people except through
a dynamic of domination and extraction. Roman soldiers
took resources and labor from Israel's territory to funnel
power and wealth across the sea to Rome.

Jesus was not a farmer, but he was intimate with the
land. The Spirit led him to wild and lonely places to pray.

What did he do for forty days, hungry, in the desert? Did he draw in the sand, look for shapes in the clouds? I don't think Jesus's time in gardens and on lakes, in deserts and on mountains, was at all incidental to his ministry. Amidst all the pressures of his life, he must have met God and himself in a unique way, out there, to keep returning. I imagine him filling up on peace and deep breaths in a meadow or cave, in order to pour out again once he returned to the crowds.

One of the earliest stories Judaism and Christianity share is a creation story about a God who looks at the world and its soil and sees that it needs tending. So God carefully, lovingly, playfully even, forms the first human out of the soil itself. God calls the human *Adam*, naming him after the soil—*adamah*—from which he was birthed, the substance that shapes him and that will continue to sustain his life. God plants a garden and sculpts more animals out of the clay beneath God's feet. God is always bringing life and art out of the dirt, and teaching the first humans to do the same.

I think Jesus knew the soil as kin. He must have heard often—after the "love your enemies" bit, or the Beatitudes, maybe—that his ideas wouldn't work in the "real world." *But which real world?* he seemed always to say. *When was the last time you sat and watched a river go by, or met a bird, or even considered the lilies?*

In many ways, the "realest" world we are connected to is the world of our most immediate bodily needs—our animal selves. If Jesus's incarnation mattered, it's because however ethereally "spiritual" and wise he may have been, he was, in equal proportion, material: sunburnt and squishy, dusty and desirous. I think he knew he belonged to the earth. I think he navigated empire's cities and its egos with the humble confidence of one who knows himself to be Spirit and dirt and blood.

————

In writing this chapter, I've discarded page after page of overthinking, over-researched, overexplaining attempts to contain all the complexity of what it means to take environmental health seriously as a predictor of our own health. I want to get it right; I want to do justice to the truth of how our bodies, our communities, our economies, and our ecosystems all overlap and interact. I want us to reimagine this earth, not as our container but as our home; not as a sphere of raw material to be extracted but as an infinitely complex and creative being in her own right. I want to put words to what it means to live a creaturely life.

More than that, though, in writing and rewriting I've wanted to present us with an "answer." We are wondrous, fragile, body-bound creatures, but we are also clever and powerful beings who bear great responsibility for what we have done to this planet in the past—and how we could live with her in the future. I want to be able to say how we are going to live up to the beauty of this earth and the stewardship to which we are called. Somewhere in my not-quite-conscious mind, I think I am going to write my way into "the solution" for neatly untangling all the destruction and carefully fixing everything.

I'm constantly tempted to say something like, "We should all get more curious and more involved with our food, from soil to plate." But such a statement ignores the fact that "we all" don't have choices or answers about our food available to us. "We all" shouldn't necessarily *have* to become cooks, gardeners, or farmer's market aficionados in order to procure nourishing food from ethical sources. And that's not a magic fix, anyway: some things about our food system will never change due to individual consumer choices, but depend on legislation or industry standards.

Besides, I haven't even lived up to my own "shoulds," let alone those I'd proclaim over everyone else. I haven't always maintained my strict ethical meat standards. I forget to even consider the provenance of my food when I'm at a restaurant. And only the hardiest plants have survived my several seasons of gardening. Reality is never as neat as our idyllic visions; even within my own well-resourced house, food utopia has not been achieved.

What I really mean to say, instead, is that we all *deserve to be able* to be curious about and involved with our food. It's so central to our lives and so vital to our bodies and communities, we must continue to question a world where access to a variety of nourishing food is treated as a niche market or a status symbol for the wealthy and well-educated.

We owe it to each other to support local, ethical, Black and Indigenous, or regenerative farmers and landowners, and to increase access to their products. We owe it to our kids to teach them about the ecosystems they belong to, and invite them into the work of nourishing themselves and the land. We owe it to the planet to consider major shifts on a society-wide scale so we can do less *extracting* food from the soil, and more nurturing the land and each other. We owe it to ourselves to ask why it's so hard to find the time to cook and eat good food. And we owe it to everyone who's been harmed by nutrient poverty, food apartheid, hunger, environmental destruction, environmental racism, and more, to make it a major goal of our lives together to make fresh, nutritious food available and accessible to all.

We're so far from achieving those realities that no one person can draw the map to get from here to there. So often in the past, grand schemes to fix systems like these have had such unintended consequences that they've made things worse. It's all too complex for any single person or group to understand.

But when we look to the earth herself to learn the work of repair, this complexity and the slowness of the work ahead don't seem so discouraging. Growing healthy soil, for instance, is not merely about somehow getting exactly the right amounts of certain nutrients into the ground. It takes time, seasons, and rest, while the "work" takes place invisibly among plant roots, fungi, bacteria, insects, and other animals. Humans can gently encourage these processes and nurture these organisms, too, using our own skills and technologies—but not without help, and not overnight.

Even in the microcosm of my own body, no one knew exactly how to shift my systems out of emergency mode and into a more sustainable place. We simply had to begin. At first we used drug technologies to calm the worst of the symptoms, while slowly shifting these other aspects of my life: hormone and gut support, food, stress, community. Now my only current prescriptions are for hormones, but that doesn't mean the drugs I took before were "wrong" or that I won't use them again. The matrix of things my body needs to stay healthy will probably continue to change throughout my life. Just as much as it has mattered to get that matrix "right," it has mattered to develop skills for careful and kind attention, flexibility, habit change, and endurance in continuing to care for myself.

In our sprawling, complex food systems, we're seeing all kinds of ideas and solutions for new ways of feeding people pop up at many different places. None of them—neither "ugly produce" nor school gardens nor animal welfare labeling nor locavore movements nor individual brands' commitments—is the solution to our enormous and varied food problems. But each of them is an experiment, or a stopgap, or a piece of the puzzle, and taken together, they're beginning to shift our collective awareness of what is and our imagination for what could be.

The more I study this particular system and the ways social change takes place, the more inclined I am to think it's a good thing that all these solutions are "too small" or narrow, as I've seen many of them criticized for being. To change such an enormous, interlocking system, we'll need to make a lot of mistakes, spend a lot of money, and overcome a lot of resistance from powerful interests. Each of these projects, groups, and businesses is finding its own way forward, boldly taking different approaches and risks, entering into this gigantic puzzle from one small point. They're making tiny shifts, not catastrophic ones—but just because we don't see major change today doesn't mean it's not on its way. Some of these tiny shifts are iterating, interacting, and evolving into bigger ones. Some are creating change that only seems insignificant because it is unmeasurable.

It remains to be seen how governments, farmers, scientists, distributors, restaurants, stores, consumers, and cooks will interact to tackle issues of soil health, carbon emissions and deforestation, animal welfare, and food access. We'll need resilience, creativity, and cooperation to coordinate the shifts needed to grow all of the moving pieces into a more just and equitable food system. We'll need to measure and design for life in the long term rather than profits in the short term. We'll need to imagine our agricultural, shopping, cooking, and eating lives less like machines and more like the living, breathing, vital arts, the practices and systems of care, that they are.

This reimagining and relearning won't feel like it's making a difference. The balance of power will still belong for a long time to corporations and regulators. But new ways of dreaming, talking, buying, cooking, and eating on a small scale are our most effective tools for introducing our neighbors to the need for change on a large scale. Corporations and regulators won't change their behavior until we have a collective conversation about whether the lives of people like me are important enough for change, or whether "healthy" people, themselves, are really bearing an acceptable amount of pesticides, or maybe about whether we even want to think about where our food comes from at all.

We'd have to talk about the consequences of that choice too. If environmental regulations make things more expensive, are we willing to pay? If it makes them more inconvenient, are we willing to reorganize our lives? If the thing is food, will we help our poor and working-class neighbors pay for it? These aren't things we figure out on Twitter; they're questions we struggle with in our families and neighborhoods.

The problem, the beauty, and the opportunity in the conundrum of moving from the small to the large scale is that the most difficult part of making change in a system isn't the practicalities of moving all the inputs and outputs around—even when the pieces are big and complex. The most difficult part is reimagining all the hundreds of relationships between all the pieces and people in the system. Fertilizers, herbicides, and pesticides have taken the place of relationships among crops, ecosystems, farmers, and eaters. How do we restore those relationships? How do we use our technological tools to serve them? How do we navigate the real pain, difficulty, and beauty in the process of moving from something sterile into something alive?

Such a project might seem overwhelming, but the very interconnected nature of it means you and I can start right now. It means that process begins as soon as we pay attention to, or play with, our own relationships to the world, to each other, to power, and to ourselves. It may feel like the federal legislation needed to solve a problem is out of reach, but "political will" is not some force out in the universe; it is our values and concerns. In the case of food systems, it's about my relationships with food and eating; our cultural imagination around farms, food processing, and grocery stores; your beliefs about good work, good food, and who deserves them.

The smallest experiments in doing things differently can become the signposts shouting, "Such a thing is possible!" Deep love and commitment to life in a very specific place at a very specific time will seem woefully inadequate on some days, but it is the most scalable thing on earth. After all, when I think of a deeply healthy world, I don't think of a place where everyone's body and mind are the same. I think of a world where my current version of health is allowed to belong—where my needs are accommodated and my contributions aren't overlooked—alongside hundreds and thousands of other pictures of health and healing. We don't need more laws that force conformity and efficiency onto people and communities with different needs. We need creative reimaginings that remove barriers and provide resources to the diverse ecosystem of healing solutions already springing up.

———

At the hardest times of my life, I have taken refuge in unbuilt places. As a student with high-functioning depression, I would disappear into the woods. In Boston I sought out the river and the reservoir as I wrestled with God. And when I got sick, I would stand at the edge of South Carolina, feeling the Atlantic Ocean eroding the sand beneath my feet, wondering if I would ever again stand on solid ground—but slowly coming to know that there was a reliable rhythm of rest here on the shifting sand too.

And yes: I went camping. Since my college days of fleeing to the forests and mountains, I've learned what was happening under those sanctuary canopies. Spending time in green spaces or natural environments measurably improves health outcomes and helps us regulate our overstimulated nervous systems. Our bodies and minds recognize our origins in the dirt, remembering our belonging, with the other creatures, to this home.

When I'm tempted to doubt the wisdom and wonder of my body, I bring my bare feet to meet the earth. I remember with what wisdom and grace—if also discomfort and even danger—God's creation has always met me, any time I've been humble enough to listen to it. Even in my urban backyard, remembering my own peace amid the dirt and the birds, the microbes and the towering old trees, reminds me that the honest, humble, and generous thing is to believe my body, a member of this ancient community.

Here my sublime contemplation also draws me back, gently but irresistibly, into action beyond myself. To honor this community, to stand in this soil with integrity, is not just to attend to my own healing. It is also to tell the earth's truths in places where decisions are being made about our future with her. It is to learn to be in meaningful, active solidarity with this land's rightful Indigenous caretakers. It is to return for all my life to the work of protecting the earth, of changing our lives as much as is required to repent from our failure to care for her—and it is to continually return to hear her counsel so that I *can* sustain that work for the decades it will ask of me.

I am slow, uncertain, and imperfect at this sort of engagement. Public and political activism are often fraught and exhausting. They can feel hopeless in a conservative state in an oil- and gas-hungry country. There is no manual and no welcome committee into the often tedious work of citizenship.

I bring these frustrations and failures to the Holy Spirit and the four pecan trees and the sandy soil. The wind answers in the leaves and blows through my lungs. "Who asked you," it responds, "to be speedy, certain, or perfect?"

This backyard changes from week to week, season to season, and every being who touches it takes up a different role just as often.

My own body, whom I once regarded as a static thing—one that was either working at full capacity or totally failing—is, like any other organism, a dynamic collection of systems that are forever in motion. The molecules and microbes that make up "me" will be different tomorrow than they are today; so will my life, my projects, my organizations, and my interactions with them. I'm not called to fully comprehend, freeze, describe, or manipulate any of these in all their complexity—in other words, to *control* them. Instead, I am here to meet the various circumstances and communities of my life, attend to them, cooperate with them, in full knowledge that I can't control anything or guarantee any outcome. I can only guarantee that I am committed to staying present to the never-ending processes of evolution and change.

Most of us have much more to offer by letting go than by seizing the illusion of control. It is not ours to fix, win, or be (or pretend to be) the perfect activist. Sometimes it is ours to witness, sometimes to write, sometimes to march, sometimes to babysit or set a table, sometimes to argue or dance or pray, and sometimes to love and trust others enough to rest. It is not ours to *accomplish* God's peace, justice, and Wholeness.

It is ours to show up imperfectly to where it is already taking shape.

10

FROM DISCONNECTION TO WHOLENESS

I once sat in a required college class slumping in one of those desks-attached-to-the-chair, skimming a long introductory textbook chapter about defining "health." At the time, I found this incredibly pedantic. Of course it seemed important to acknowledge that health has multiple dimensions: physical, mental, relational, and so on. But beyond that, it also seemed self-evident to me that you'd know health when you saw it. Health is when you don't have to think about your health. Health is not-disease, health is functioning, health is normalcy.

From that perspective, I'm not sure I should be writing a book about health and healing. By that common, intuitive definition, health and chronic illness must be mutually exclusive; a synonym for chronic illness would be "perpetual unhealth."

I don't exactly feel the need to claim healthy status. I don't believe healthy people are any better, more worthy, or more deserving than sick people—whether their sickness is a genetic fluke or the direct result of alternating cigarettes, beer, and ice cream for years at a time. No one deserves to suffer. We too often create false dichotomies between "healthy" and "unhealthy" people, activities, or foods in order to imply that some people are more virtuous and some more expendable than others. I won't play into that game by trying to worm my way onto the healthy side.

Still, as I wrote this book I realized that as much as I think of myself as chronically ill, I also feel myself to be chronically healing. Not healing as in returning to an uncompromised state of perfection, but healing as an activity of resisting destruction and decay, of choosing kindness, nourishment, and self-support. Others might call it "disease management," but it is more than a series of steps for maintaining a semblance of control. It's a way of life that offers time, resources, and honor to the body and to the care it needs. It's tending to the relationships—between body and soul, between self and community, between my cells and those of the land—that constitute sustenance and resilience, but that our burnout culture constantly frays.

I witness my friends with mental illness, who've survived trauma, or who live with disabilities also creating this healing way for themselves. We are both sick, damaged, or abnormal, and finding our own way to our own kind of health. We are experts at attending to what is needed, what is good and pleasurable, what resources we can use creatively, what our bodies and minds have to say about our lives and the world around us—and often, doing it all over again from scratch every day. We are experts at healing. This is how we survive.

When we even *begin* to let go of the false binary between "health" (perfection? functioning? productivity?) and unhealth, we discover that a large majority of us actually live our lives in this in-between place. Most people have some "issue," wound, illness, weakness, or insufficiency that haunts us, and for which we too often feel ashamed. Most of us would benefit immensely if the world were a little kinder and more accessible—even if that meant the world became a little less productive. Most of us have let ourselves be convinced that our "defect" or limitation puts us beyond the pale of normalcy, makes us less-than in some way, must be compensated for (but not accommodated).

When we add up all the burdens, illnesses, mental health needs, neurodivergences, and disabilities in the world, we discover that it's the rare person who isn't regularly excluded from the "normal," "healthy," or nondisabled standard. But if that picture of perfect health is supposed to be a baseline—the way we're all assumed to be able to operate—how is it that the vast majority of us feel we can only aspire to it? True, some people hide their weakness or manage their disease well enough to pretend, because that's how you're supposed to get by or get ahead, but in the end, they still know pain and precarity. They ultimately belong more in this both/and world than in the world that renders them invisible.

I believe, if we acknowledged how many of us are both sick or wounded *and* healing, far fewer of us would feel the need to pretend. We could start to dismantle the narrative that health is some kind of prize for doing all the right things, or that illness is an inconvenient exception to the rule. We could face the facts, that illness is a part of every human life, and chronic or mental illness is part of most. Even those who don't suffer from a disorder have limitations; you don't need a diagnosis in order to honor your own uniqueness and finitude.

If we collectively paused to listen to illness, perhaps we could learn from chronically ill people the art of living sustainably.

————

The pandemic languishes; it presses in on me like the summer sun piercing the curtains from early morning to the slow-falling night; it seeps into my lungs like muggy air. It flattens me into surrender to hot stillness, to a planetary sort of inevitability, to daydreams of somewhere else.

I don't want to "be with my emotions" anymore. I don't want to rage against the person or group I blame today. I can't scheme or strategize anymore. I don't think about when this will end; I don't imagine how to help anyone; I don't wish for anything. Instead, I look to the next hour, as if I am a fruit fly. I eat when I'm hungry. I text friends when I'm lonely. I work for a few minutes when I'm bored. I am in despair, all the time.

In principle, I don't believe in despair. In principle, I believe in being faithful to a calling with humility and trust. I've taken to pretending those principles actually make sense to me: I write my writings and clean my kitchen. And the whole time, I am quietly broken; I am the withering plants blasted in the garden by too much sun and then too much rain.

"Move like you are in water," says the YouTube yoga instructor, and I think this is what I am doing all the time, swimming anew in incomprehension. I am out of energy for statistics, R-values, or diagrams showing how breath vapor makes invisible, deadly clouds out of speech and song.

I cannot calculate any more risk, but I can feel fear in my guts when I go out, so I stay home.

The world's disease is flaring. And if the world were a single fellow sick person, maybe I could rock them in my lap when they started to panic; maybe I could say, "I know. I know it hurts." I would make them a cup of tea and wrap them in blankets and they would rest, and later, maybe, we would ask their body questions.

Where is the hurt?

Where is the exhaustion?

When fear and loneliness ooze up to you with their lies, where have they crept up from?

When you pull them close and don't let them go, what truths do you learn that they were hiding?

What feels good?

What one thing feels necessary?

What if bravery is a soft and tender thing?

What is there to lose from being kind?

But the world is not a person, and my questions burn away under the sun like mid-morning clouds, and if the cicadas' chattering chant is an answer, I cannot understand.

If the sick person were me, on the other hand, the questions would be a little more straightforward. Years of deep listening, doctor co-pays, and self-experimentation, and weeks buried in research have put me a few steps down the line from *Where does it hurt?* Instead, the questions are decidedly practical. When the world's falling apart, it's,

Do you have energy for a twenty-minute walk? No? A five-minute walk?

Have you eaten a vegetable?

Taken your meds?

Called a friend?

Can you just rest today?

Here is a heating pad.
Here is a hammock.
Here is a voice of gentleness.

Because even though a flare feels like—can be—an emergency, I know by now that it's weeks in the making. Weeks of drift away from nourishing food habits, or of stubbornly forgetting my supplements and meds, or of stress that I haven't released having overwhelmed me. In the face of my pain, none of these tiny actions feels like a solution, but they are the building blocks of a healing way of life deep and strong enough to contain the great force of autoimmunity. Even a five-minute walk is a beginning.

Without the privilege of steady care, though, experiencing acute symptoms of chronic illness can feel like panic. Poverty, misdiagnosis, denial, or a lack of any number of supports can lead to a cycle where chronic illness is only treated when it's most unbearable, while it slowly worsens over time in between emergencies.

Over time, it can lead to the kind of despair that makes addiction feel like delivery into gentler arms. It's too hard to hurt without knowing when or if it will be over. It is too much to live with hope and trust only to see them crushed all over again.

But when we turn toward the chronic illness of our world, we too often try and force ourselves into this very pattern. Wildfires in the West are acute symptoms of the chronic condition of climate change. Police murders, of White supremacy and colonizer violence. Crime and addiction, of preventable poverty. When we respond by engaging only in reactive politics and not in long-term structural solutions to our world's deepest wounds; when we're pressured into "productivity" in the face of pain; when we entertain a toxic positivity that won't allow us to be prepared for the next flare, we are not engaging in healing or care at all—only triage.

In reality, the acute symptoms of a chronic condition call for *both* emergency action to lessen the distress *and* long-term changes to address root causes and support overall healing. But without competent, holistic care, we're not able to face all of it. We bounce between ever-worsening acute episodes and ever more drastic short-term interventions.

After five years of illness, a flare can still feel like a summons to drastic action; but in reality it is, first of all, an invitation to re-grounding and recentering in deep, focused attention to mundane habits of care. Of course, years ago adopting these habits was a life-changing challenge. Now, the fact that they feel frustratingly small doesn't make them any less powerful.

Colonial culture—ever focused on the future, ever in pursuit of "growth"—actively dismisses and demeans this kind of work. It celebrates inventors and "pioneers," philanthropists and political fixers who claim to have grand solutions for us. Faithful acts of care and maintenance disappear, and we tell our most essential workers to stay invisible.

So when we are faced with a wicked disease, a humanitarian crisis, or a racial reckoning, we are primed to cast about for hyped-up heroes and grand gestures. But the work of real, clear-eyed attention actually calls us to the quiet and quotidian, to actions whose very power lies in their mundane repeatability, to the kind of radical change so deep it is imperceptible for weeks or months or years.

When it hurts so much, we only want the pain to stop, and it's massively overwhelming to hear that so much will be required of us. We see a list of tasks and chores rolling out indefinitely in front of us, *just to get back to normal.*

I didn't stop feeling stressed out and put-upon by all the care my body needed until I accepted that the point was to never go back to normal. Even if I could do that, my experiences had already changed who I was. Since I couldn't—and since "normal" had made me sick to begin with—my task was not to cram all these requirements and activities in alongside my old life, but to reorient my life now around practices of healing.

This is the same long, boring, and beautiful discipline we must practice when it comes to the sicknesses of our society. Not only to march in the streets—or feel guilty for not marching in the streets—when things are unconscionably bad, but to reclaim and redefine engaged citizenship as something we can rebuild together, with slow and steady care. We will have to let go of "normal"—even when it's painful—in order to make room to reorient our lives around practices of healing together.

————

When I first imagined writing this book, it was a book about the many evils I had to unlearn in order to heal with a disease caused by disorders that afflict us all. I wrote about extraction and colonialism, White supremacy and patriarchy. "Lyndsey's body is a prophet!" cried one friend workshopping an early draft.

These were words I'd used myself. After so long ignoring her myself, I wanted my body's rage and desperation to be heard.

But as I wrote on, I discovered that my body's prophecies came in many forms. She is no stranger to the language of desperation and rage; but she also communicates in registers of desire, pleasure, rest, and relief; she knows the music of sorrow and sharing; she is fluent in limits, seasons, para-doxes, relationality, and never-ending change.

For a while I learned from my body what needed to change; more recently her insistent schooling has been in *how* to go about doing it. Those lessons have become the true shape of this book.

Some people will wish I'd written the first version. There's not nearly enough *demand* here, they might say. These ills can't be remedied without mass, disciplined, grueling and risky action. All this individual, inner change can do noth-ing without movements to effect systemic reform. These ideas could even be *dangerous* if they delay or distract from taking action.

I agree with these warnings. I agree with them so much that I've taken them as a given throughout this book. I trust readers to understand that, just as I couldn't furrow my brow, describe my pain, and expect healing to follow, nei-ther can we take concern or discomfort about injustice to be the same as action.

I've also spent enough time in community organizing work and in friendship with other activists to witness the damage caused by a false dichotomy between personal or small-scale transformation and systemic change. It is not my experience that people in movement spaces are in danger of attending too much to our pain. Instead, many of us are run-ning from, reenacting, or brandishing our wounds as a way to avoid facing, tending, processing, and integrating them.

This is not to say that only "healed" people can do this work. On the contrary, our movements must center on those who face injustice and discrimination *daily*—who are most deeply acquainted with the chronic nature of our collective disorder. In order to do that, we must enter into daily practices of healing and healing together. This healing justice is a movement lineage tracing to the Kindred South-ern Healing Justice Collective: "Our movements themselves have to be healing," said Black and Indigenous founder Cara Page, "or there is no point to them."

This means embracing a both/and approach to healing and health: recognizing that individual health is a precarious illusion without systemic supports for collective health—but neither can we claim to pursue Wholeness while asking each other (or ourselves) to subordinate or sacrifice individual health to a future vision of collective healing. Instead, we must reject a false dichotomy between self and community, inward-out and outward-in, present and future healing. Wherever we find personal healing and integration, we build better relationships and healthier communities. Wherever we learn more just and loving habits in our families, we learn to interrupt unjust patterns in wider organizations. When we find ways to work together without reverting to capitalist cultures of using ourselves and others, the things we create together become far stronger, more sustainable, and more adaptable. Tending to habits and qualities like rest, responsibility, boundaries, and relationships of humility, honesty, and respect are not distractions from or accessories to the project of systemic healing and Wholeness. They *are* the material of systemic healing and Wholeness.

I learned this in my own life with chronic illness. It booted me out of my conquer-and-control approach to life and into a place where I had to make friends with all the things I'd once considered irrelevant at best, and enemies at worst: things like uncertainty. Bodily feelings and desires. Soul emotions and longings. Interdependence. Imagination and art. Limitation and failure. Dependence on the land. Rest, connection, and joy.

These may sound like spiritual goods or personal growth qualities, but they are also an alternative path for being strategic about reaching goals and changing the world. They are not only "nice" or moral; they are effective tools when we learn to practice them together. Along the way of learning to reimagine career, advocate for social justice, and grow community alongside this healing journey, I've made lots of friends and learned from many scholars who are reimagining power. They're finding ways to create real shifts in the world without dominating and controlling each other, extracting resources from land or people, or flattening difference for the sake of efficiency. For them, lost pieces of our humanity—like our bodies and emotions, or creativity and spirituality—are not merely accessories to their work; they are its essence.

That's not to say that tools like technology, legislation, and planning for efficiency are wrong. But, like pharmaceutical drugs and lab tests, they should be used to serve humans, not as the external benchmarks of success which humans must serve. They're allowed to be adapted and adaptable, not built into a rigid plan that can't change. They enter into the strategic process at the end, after people have decided on the how and the why. When we make our tools into ends instead of means, we may think we're trying to chart the most direct course to a goal of prosperity or justice; but we actually constrain our vision of what is possible, what is moral, what contributes to Wholeness.

On the other hand, when we accept that we cannot control or predict the outcomes of our work, but channel more intentionality into centering our processes on people, we may find our vision expanding. New possibilities for outcomes, multiple paths to accomplishing our goals, or a range of responses to the unexpected present themselves when we take care of each other, embrace creativity, and resist the short-term thinking that capitalism has trained us in.

In the same way, I can't control or predict the outcomes of my disease, but in some ways I've become *more* prepared for the future as a result. I've learned how to make flexible plans and build resilient supports into them. I'm not baffled by "failure" or helplessness when problems arise. I'm practiced in the art of prioritizing.

And I have discovered, by painful trial and error, that I rise and fall during my struggles by the quality of my tiny, boring, even tedious habits during better times. Regular yoga practice, investment in friendships, and enjoyable cooking habits *before* a flare hits can make the difference between a flare that levels me for months and a body supported to slow down and then repair more quickly.

Another practice I've discovered is to attend to my joy, laughter, liberation, and peace as closely as to my pain. When overwhelmed by fatigue and fear, it's easy to see how dis-ease operates on a self-perpetuating feedback loop, consuming me in the process. Yet I've also experienced how the courage to be attentive and vulnerable to joy can spiral and spread in the opposite direction. I am learning, even when preoccupied by pain or fear, to find real rest in entering fully into even momentary experiences of beauty, wonder, connection, and joy. I remember that I am more than my pain, and the world is more than broken. As adrienne maree brown says, "What we pay attention to grows."

———

In an effort to pay better attention, I did eventually take up meditation: brushing up against the unfamiliar experience of stillness, breathing in and breathing out.

At times, when I've imagined breathing into the great web of life, I've seen myself as an indistinguishable node among nodes in a network, or as a hollow vessel through which the rest of the world could simply flow in and out. In some ways, this mirrors the feminist concept of Eros, "the energy of all relationship." It's a beautiful, powerful, and humbling thing to know ourselves constituted by so many others.

But Eros is also more than that. To claim our belonging to the web of life, we must *participate* in it; we must rise up to meet it. None of us is an empty vessel. We are quite full, of embodied experiences, longings and joys, particular loves and particular relationships. To take Eros seriously is to know that it can only be fully accessed through all of ourselves. We have each been entrusted with one person to tend, love, and forgive for our entire lives; taking up our place in Eros means embracing that person—our truest self—and inviting them with courage and compassion to show up to the dance. We are not merely *in* so many systems; we *make up* the systems. Every time we feed, nurture, or challenge ourselves, we are also deeply loving the world.

Theologian Rita Nakashima Brock calls this self—the self who resides among body, mind, spirit, and emotions all at once, the deeply vulnerable and thus deeply powerful, the fathomless, often-forgotten, so very beloved self—"heart." She speaks of Eros as "knowing by heart," as a parallel for the Hebrew word *daath* for "know," which means to know with all of oneself.

The Hebrew and Greek words often translated in the Bible as "heart" in a metaphorical sense come from the literal heart. It is the innermost, central organ of the body, connected so inextricably to all the other organs, whose beating rhythm may be hidden but cannot lie.

Jesus knew by heart, Brock says. He moved through the world in community, growing his ministry alongside others and ultimately entrusting it entirely to them. He was not a lofty, lonely figure harboring an otherworldly well of magical power. Jesus drew on the God-given power of the dance of life, showing up fully—in great courage and great vulnerability. He met others in the space of their own hearts, inviting them to return to their fullest selves and to the truth of the communion of the world.

To take Wholeness seriously is to attend to the hidden, Spirit-empowered energy of Eros. And to recognize the sacredness of heart, body, and breath is also to grieve and to act when these are being stolen by the sicknesses of our world. Environmental injustice destroys species and chokes lungs; Black communities cry out "I can't breathe"; COVID-19 is allowed to rampage through our cities and towns, disproportionately affecting disabled, elderly, poor, Native, Black, and Brown communities.

When our neighbor is sick, it is rarely up to any individual to ensure the outcome of healing for them. But we can move toward them instead of looking away, offer a hand or a ride, check back in again later. Like the women at the foot of the cross, like the Christ who saw the suffering, like the Spirit who comes alongside, we can choose to stay.

Jesus stays with us as one of the breathless and brokenhearted. Rome disabled God, this God of power-through-vulnerability. He loved the world, and the world killed him. When we are breathless and brokenhearted, abandoned and sick, God is with us. The life of God with us was a life of radical solidarity with our embodied, interconnected human existence, with the poor and the outcast (whom Brock calls the "brokenhearted"). He showed us how to re-knit Wholeness where it was severed by sin, one broken heart at a time. In the midst of cruel, heartless empire, here was God's kin-dom come.

I still don't think Jesus has ever "lived in" anyone's heart. But if he could draw out our truest, hidden, and hurting selves; if he could meet us in our humanity, imperfect bodies and minds, emotions and spirits and all; if he could restore people to a community healed by the remembered presence of love and power of the Holy Spirit; maybe he does return *us* to live courageously, in and by our hearts.

In meditation, I meet my heart, my body, and Spirit all over again. *This* breath in *this* moment in *this* body is the place where I am tethered to the natural world, a habitat I once thought of as a place I "visited" but now know myself to be inseparable from. I befriend my animal body. I come to know her restlessnesses, her wants and warnings. When my bare feet meet my weed-strewn grass, they recognize kin in this chaotic symphony of soil.

There are still times when my "self-care" regimen feels . . . regimental, a long list of tiresome tasks I'd rather ignore. But the more I come to inhabit my body, to truly dwell in my own experience of myself, the less my daily walks, yoga, pills, diet, and all the rest seem like imposed chores. Instead, they're simply the things I hunger for—even part of what it means to be *me.*

I watch my houseplants turn toward the sun. I see the roots of my pecan trees seeking out stability, nutrients, and their favorite fungi. I stop on my walk so the dog can snort and roll in her favorite long, soft grass. And I think again that these are my mentors, never ashamed of their own needs but unhesitatingly answering what draws them.

And the more I say yes to my own desires, the more I make time, the more I choose consistent care over emergency fixes—the more time I spend with my heart and God's Spirit—the more this body is safe to speak to me.

I would like to say that from this place I've experienced some flash of insight or great Knowing about what I should do For Justice. Isn't that the kind of neat line we'd like to draw between inner and outer, personal and communal healing? But I haven't found the perfect role in the perfect organization, been seized by a single issue, or become a yoga teacher or a therapist. Instead, I've been led to lend a hand to organizations run by people I trust. I've tried to support the many activists, farmers, teachers, pastors, therapists, and yoga teachers I know and love. And I've sat and prayed in witness, in grief, in vigil, in acceptance of a stubbornly sick world. This planet is changing, and I cannot slow or stop it. I am still learning to meet it with kindness and grace.

In the reality of this changing planet, adrienne maree brown draws on an art installation by artist collective Complex Movements to describe how we need our work to have a *mycelial* element. Mycelia are the thread-like strands that make up most fungi, including the vast networks of tiny filaments that wend throughout soils and funnel nutrients and messages between plants. Plant roots and fungi have coevolved for so long that in many cases, the two organisms can be distinguished, but can't be separated. Mycelia also help metabolize dead and even toxic material in the environment. They make up an utterly indispensable, nearly invisible connective tissue of forest ecosystems that was almost totally overlooked by science until the twentieth century.

Like scientists who are too busy studying plants to ever bother with soils and fungi—and therefore, fundamentally misunderstand plants—we don't have formal channels or even vocabulary in many of our organizations for recognizing the work that takes place underground. But those who make art out of refuse, those who create and maintain hospitable space for connection among others, those who do the invisible, repetitive tasks and the hidden work of healing are doers of justice. We are tending to the very threads of relationship that constitute Wholeness.

CONCLUSION

We are bombarded with information, news, and opinions from the moment we wake until they chase us into our dreams. In the isolation of the pandemic, we've turned ever more often to the Internet to gain some sense of purchase, of connection, of belonging. We've had to try and piece together a working understanding of virology, epidemiology, and public health from our kitchen tables, because so many institutions have failed us so profoundly. Trying to make sense of the systems that surround us, to know our place in them, and to be agents of justice and Wholeness within them feels more overwhelming than ever.

With every chapter of this book I've wanted to gather more data, read more history, determine where the healthcare or economy or food system is going, and tell you what to do about it. But this is not a book about how to wrest back control over our lives and the world—as if "doing the right thing" would entitle us to such. This is not a book about any outcome at all. This book is about living, here and now, in a crumbling empire.

At the ends of books like these, we expect to find hope. For much of my life, I refused to talk about hope. The "hope" week of Advent was the time I most consistently wondered whether my religion wasn't all a pack of comforting lies. I never found a definition of hope that I liked. The closest I came was an appreciation for those who admitted that they needed something like it to shore up their determination to go down swinging.

I've spent much of the pandemic grappling with the fact that many people would rather die an excruciating death, alone, than admit that their fate is bound up with that of their neighbor. Whether these people are depraved or just deluded doesn't really matter. I still lie awake wondering—if we cannot take a straightforward path to escape clear and present danger to ourselves, how will we ever save each other from all our self-imposed harms?

The truth is, if I knew an answer, I'd be making a lot more money to write this book. The truth is, when I ask God this question, I don't get a clear or comforting reply.

But ever since I got sick in 2016, I've gotten to learn from folks in the Poor People's Campaign and at Two Rivers Church, the scrappy survivors and allies of the Lee University Affirming Alum Collective, the activists in my neighborhood at Fresh Future Farm and the disabled people in my life. They've taught me a hope beyond some blithe assurance that my preferred outcome is imminent. I find a far more honest hope, a quiet but scrappy hope, blooming in the most unlikely places among these friends and mentors. Hope finds me, not in clinging to one version of my favorite imagined future, but in being present to what is here now. Hope is not trusting that God has to make things turn out the way I want, but that God is with us already.

It's like this, after all, when you're chronically ill. Having an incurable illness doesn't doom you to hopelessness. It means life will be different. It means grieving the old life, one you hadn't known was ending. But eventually, it also means finding unexpected sources of joy and purpose squarely within the once-dreaded parameters of this unlooked-for life.

A few weeks ago, I lay on an acupuncturist's table trying to explain why I felt so stuck.

I was there to treat my physical body, but our conversation had turned to life, stuck-ness, and grief. I noticed that my breath would get stuck in my chest. I felt weighed down by a creeping accumulation of disappointments, small losses, and long sorrows. Heading into year three of the pandemic, I found myself wondering if there was anything other than sadness and disconnection in store for us any time soon. Tears rolled down the sides of my face as I struggled to explain. And if I couldn't fully describe where all this was coming from, I didn't have the courage to say, *How could I wade into the waters of grief? What if there was no bottom?*

"Do you have space in your schedule for this?" Christina asked—to reach beyond a few tears and release the tide?

I wasn't entirely sure if I did or not. But I'd felt increasingly as though this grief was slowly suffocating me, like as long as I couldn't access it, it was seeping into everything I did, turning things gray, and creating a fog between me and others.

I took a beat. When do you schedule a descent into the abyss? "Yes."

The first needles went normally: a little ache or tingle that soon subsided.

Then: "Grief can constrict our chests," Christina said. "Breathe in . . . breathe out." The final needle went in below my sternum. *Ouch.* The next breath in—*OUCH.* What was happening? Christina looked unconcerned as she placed her palm on my shoulder. I breathed again: *OUCH,* but bearable.

"Your job for the next twenty minutes is to breathe deeply, in and out," Christina said like always. She turned the lights off and left the room.

Ouch.

Now more tears were falling down my face. I *wanted* to follow my deep-breathing instructions; I *needed* those sad little huffy shuddering breaths you take when you're crying; but with every single inhale, my chest and stomach would rise and this needle would sink in. I felt my body trying to inhale into every part of itself *except* the very center of my lungs, to avoid disturbing this needle, to skirt the edges of the pain.

Breathe.

But it hurts.

I opened my lungs fully into the sensation anyway. It hurt.

It hurts to breathe.

I want to not hurt. I want to not breathe.

But this is your breath. It is the only breath you have. This is your life.

Sometimes it just hurts.

Now I was sobbing. Now I was enveloped in the churning waters, in the pain of grief that my body had been trying to protect me from. All the small hurts and terrible fears and global losses of pandemic life; all the months of infertility now accumulating into years; all the things I could not fix for my family members; the years of life and the love for the world that now felt stolen by COVID-19—I'd wanted to just keep going, and my body had helped me hide from them.

My chest had slowly constricted to protect my softest self. By not breathing fully, to get around the hurt, my body felt less vulnerable. I'd unconsciously tried to avoid the bracing bravery of openness by using less and less of my airways, and living less and less of my life.

Now that I'd been given help in letting grief make itself known, it overtook everything else in me. There was a loosening, an opening, a softening in my chest, but there wasn't a bottom to the grief.

I just found myself, after a long time in the churning depths, slowly treading water and then floating on my back, gray fog gone, a faint ache in my chest letting me know I was alive.

———

Maybe there is no bottom. Maybe we won't save the planet and save ourselves. Maybe those with warped souls and death wishes really are too powerful for the rest of us to make change. Maybe the disease gets worse and the pain doesn't end. I don't believe real hope is possible unless we fully face these potential futures. In fact, refusal to even look clearly at them is at the root of much of the fear-driven hate we're seeing around us.

What I call hope in my own life is the possibility that even in such a worst-case scenario, there are still love and joy, pleasure, connection, and even peace to be pursued. Hope for me is the memory of ancestors who lived through the slow implosion of their worlds and still found pockets of life-giving love, community, and creativity. Hope is the sense that the work of making change alongside my neighbors, and of growing communities that practice the art of endurance, is the best work I can think of—whether or not our ultimate goals always succeed.

If all our catastrophes are decades in the making, there's a strange kind of pragmatic peace in accepting that they will be at least as long in the unmaking. It's good to realize that the kind of drastic and immediate change we wish for—however overdue it may objectively be—feels impossible because it *is* impossible. We don't have the resources to accomplish it; we don't have the systemic infrastructure to navigate it; we don't have the physical and emotional strength to cope with it.

But when we expand our time horizon; when we increase the profound depths at which we are willing to experience transformation; when we take seriously a commitment to a lifetime of action via sustainable means; then we discover that we have an abundance of what we need, and the capacity to grow more of it. Even better, we can honor the need for "resistance" while also recognizing that "changing the world" is far more than that. We encounter the joyful task of discovering what we are *for*, and even the possibility that fostering it might become our most profound, powerful, and winsome argument for change.

Nate and I have made hard choices about our lives in the face of my disease. And we continue to do so as we look at our lives in the context of the changing wider world. We have no delusions that we can live far from family, chase down career success, participate in deep community with our neighbors, push for justice, maintain a big house in hurricane territory, raise children, do right by our parents as they age, and care for ourselves amidst ongoing trauma all at once. To the extent that we once defined success as somehow doing it all, we have to grieve our previous visions of the future. In the real future, we may need to move closer to (or move in with) family and friends. We may need to reevaluate career trajectories or family planning decisions. We may need to choose our roles and our seasons in activism or nonprofit work with care. We may even find at times that simply caring for our neighbors, or for our own families, is all the "ministry" we can faithfully do.

And, in the face of great uncertainty, we've also grown more committed to the joy and connectedness that's available to us now, and that will sustain us through the best case or the worst. I mean the garden and the neighborhood group and all that, sure. But also, there's nothing like an unpredictable, systemic vascular illness to help you decide now is the right time to book the tickets to stand by the Adriatic Sea.

For me, it is hopeful to recognize that these massive-to-us but also mundane and pragmatic life choices matter much more than taking in all the fear, pain, and anger of today's news story. They are facilitating a way of life that is creatively and lovingly counter-empire, in whatever ways make sense for us and our family. They are the ongoing care for the chronic condition, which we trust will make the acute symptoms less destructive. Being committed to relationships of solidarity, mutual aid, and care—and slowly discerning how to shape our lives around those—has the potential to free us from the nagging sense that justice is something we are simply tacking on or fitting in.

This is a humbler and kinder way of justice; this is the unglamorous, but surprisingly joyful, way of faithfulness. We are not always called to join every worthy organization, but we are always called to know our neighbors and support the leaders we hope to see succeed. We are not always called to do Great Things for The World, but we are always called to grow our capacity to do hard things with integrity. We are not always called to achieve "ally perfection," but we are always called to apologize, learn, and change when we make mistakes. We are not always called to make things turn out alright in the end, but we are always called to grow our relationships with other vulnerable people so that we know how to care for them whether things turn out alright or not. We are not always called to "lead" by taking responsibility for more and more; we are always called to invite each other to both lead and follow by contributing each person's own unique perspectives and gifts.

Precisely because these humbler habits, these slower ways of making change, these countercultural relationships are not always Instagrammable, they can actually ask more from seasoned leaders and overachievers than a big, draining, accolade-accumulating project does. They go against the grain of our hierarchical organizations, our hustle mentalities, and our unwritten status scorecards. Instead, in order to commit to a steadier and more interdependent pursuit of Wholeness and justice, we have to distribute power, prestige, and resources more equitably among our communities and organizations, allowing more people to more fully participate. In order to make our movements into healing places, we have to "skill up" at naming and repairing harm and we have to elevate those who are healing and those who heal them. In order to keep our work sustainable and invite more people into it, we have to make art, enjoyment, beauty, and celebration inseparable parts of the work itself. While we may have to struggle against "enemies" to create change, justice is not a prize we can win. It is something we must continually create for and with each other, with the help and healing of the Holy Spirit.

And still, none of it will ever be "enough." Not enough to change the world; not even enough to simply make up for the harm caused by our own complicity with systemic sin. My body will never be cured; the world will not be repaired. Healing goes on, and life continues to hurt.

But we are not here on earth to add up our lives to some cosmic math of "enough." Wholeness, real Wholeness, is so much more than such a bare hope.

We are here to lean ever deeper into the mysteries that defy our usual conceptions of that math. We are here to experience wonder at the many systems, ecosystems, and relationships that draw us into their dance, and to revel in connection with each other. We're here to make terrible mistakes and experience fearsome griefs. We are here to pray, and march, and comfort, and breathe, and spew coffee across the room laughing, and to discover that they're all the same thing.

We're here to know the God who was wounded and the God who heals, every day, all over again.

ACKNOWLEDGMENTS

All books are lived before they are written, and all works of art ultimately owe their existence to entire communities. First books, too, are almost always the products of combined hard work, luck, and privilege, and many deserving ones never make it to print. By far my greatest stroke of luck has been in knowing these kind and clever people, who have helped me live and helped me write.

Hannah, Erin, Laurel, Bethany, Olivia, Holly, Nicole, Brittany, Micky, Ty, Brittany, Taryn, Kenya, Elizabeth, Kanani, Katie, Sarah, Matt, KJ, and all my chronically ill friends: I owe you this book and I owe you my healing. You have never made me feel like Sick Woman, but you've also never allowed me to live without hope. If this list included my mentally ill friends, it would run way off the page, but you, too, have shown me how to live bravely and with love. Thank you for holding me up and showing me how beautiful we are. Thank you for living by heart with me.

Thank you to the Collegeville Institute and my writing teachers there: Enuma Okoro, Jonathan Wilson-Hartgrove, Dr. Chanequa Walker-Barnes, and Dr. Lauren Winner. I cannot overstate the value of your workshops in my life, my writing, and my writing life. Your work is resonating in the world long after it's formally ended. I'm still in awe just typing your names! Thank you for teaching and tending the writer in me.

To Keely, my agent: Your help on this proposal turned these ideas into a book. More than that, your enthusiastic support of this small-platform idealist kept me writing when I might have walked away. Thank you for believing in this book and finding it a home.

To Lisa, my editor: Thank you for loving my words more than my Instagram numbers, helping a first-time author through, and keeping me in integrity/out of embarrassment. It's been so joyful to learn from you.

To Kara, Lana, Sarah, and Olivia, and the whole "In the Thick of It" writing group: Your comments on my early draft were utterly invaluable in making this book even the least bit readable. I also printed them out and dragged them everywhere long after implementing your advice, because your care and enthusiasm for this book made writing feel so much less lonely. Thank you for accompanying me.

To Erin and Christina: Your competent, compassionate, balanced healthcare has utterly changed and possibly saved my life.

To the Sippin' Sisters: You know we deserve our own whole-ass book. Thank you for drawing me in, drawing me out, and teaching me so, so much of what is here through your love and your lives.

To the fire group: What a dream come true. When I think of being drawn toward goodness by pleasure and joy, I think of Friday nights.

To Miya: You're the best helper! What a good girl!

To Mommy and Daddy: Thank you for teaching me how to advocate for myself. Thank you for believing me when I said I was sick. Thank you for gathering me again and again. Thank you for teaching me that perfect attendance is bullshit.

To Nate: At times I didn't know how to write you into this book because I struggled to communicate just how caring, understanding, kind, self-sacrificial, compassionate, and supportive you've been throughout this unanticipated, unasked-for journey with me. You taught me everything I know about rest, self-compassion, and mutual care. I hope I get to support you in something so life-giving as unwaveringly as you've supported me in becoming a writer. Let's keep on making tater tots and making much of each other.

RESOURCES

ON SYSTEMS THINKING

brown, adrienne maree. *Emergent Strategy: Shaping Change, Changing Worlds*. Reprint edition. Chico, CA: AK Press, 2017.

Meadows, Donella H. *Thinking in Systems: A Primer*. Edited by Diana Wright. Illustrated edition. White River Junction, VT: Chelsea Green Publishing, 2008.

Schumacher, E. F. *Small Is Beautiful: Economics as if People Mattered*. New York: HarperPerennial, 1989.

ON BODIES IN CONTEXT

Copeland, Mary Shawn. *Enfleshing Freedom: Body, Race, and Being*. Minneapolis: Fortress Press, 2010.

Dusenbery, Maya. *Doing Harm: The Truth About How Bad Medicine and Lazy Science Leave Women Dismissed, Misdiagnosed, and Sick*. 1st edition. New York: HarperOne, 2018.

Eiesland, Nancy L. *The Disabled God: Toward a Liberatory Theology of Disability*. First Edition. Nashville: Abingdon Press, 1994.

Hobbes, Michael. "Everything You Know About Obesity Is Wrong." *Huffington Post*. Accessed February 1, 2022. https://highline.huffingtonpost.com/articles/en/everything-you-know-about-obesity-is-wrong/.

Morgan, J. Nicole. *Fat and Faithful: Learning to Love Our Bodies, Our Neighbors, and Ourselves*. Minneapolis: Fortress Press, 2018.

Nagoski, Emily, and Amelia Nagoski. *Burnout: The Secret to Unlocking the Stress Cycle.* New York: Ballantine, 2019.

Riley, Cole Arthur. *This Here Flesh: Spirituality, Liberation, and the Stories that Make Us.* New York: Convergent, 2022.

Taylor, Sonya Renee. *The Body Is Not an Apology: The Power of Radical Self-Love.* 2nd edition. Oakland, CA: Berrett-Koehler Publishers, 2021.

Walker-Barnes, Chanequa. *Too Heavy a Yoke: Black Women and the Burden of Strength.* Illustrated edition. Eugene, OR: Cascade Books, 2014.

ON COMMUNITY AND MAKING CHANGE

Birdsong, Mia. *How We Show Up.* New York: Hachette Go, 2020.

Brock, Rita Nakashima. *Journeys by Heart: A Christology of Erotic Power.* New York: Crossroad Pub., 1988.

Harper, Lisa Sharon. *The Very Good Gospel: How Everything Wrong Can Be Made Right.* New York: WaterBrook, 2016.

hooks, bell. *All About Love: New Visions.* New York: William Morrow Paperbacks, 2018.

Kaur, Valarie. *See No Stranger: A Memoir and Manifesto of Revolutionary Love.* New York: One World, 2020.

Murthy, Vivek H. *Together: The Healing Power of Human Connection in a Sometimes Lonely World* (New York: HarperCollins, 2020).

ON VARIOUS PRACTICALITIES

Kolber, Aundi. *Try Softer: A Fresh Approach to Move Us out of Anxiety, Stress, and Survival Mode—and into a Life of Connection and Joy.* Carol Stream, IL: Tyndale House Publishers, 2020.

McKeown, Greg. *Essentialism: The Disciplined Pursuit of Less.* 1st edition. New York: Crown, 2014.

Nestor, James. *Breath: The New Science of a Lost Art.* New York: Riverhead Books, 2020.

Paul, Annie Murphy. *The Extended Mind: The Power of Thinking Outside the Brain.* Boston: Houghton Mifflin Harcourt, 2021.

Ramsey, K. J., and Kelly M. Kapic. *This Too Shall Last: Finding Grace When Suffering Lingers.* Zondervan, 2020.

Trescott, Mickey, and Angie Alt. *The Autoimmune Wellness Handbook: A DIY Guide to Living Well with Chronic Illness.* 1st edition. New York: Rodale Books, 2016.

NOTES

INTRODUCTION

"Sixty percent of adults live": Centers for Disease Control and Prevention, "Chronic Diseases in America," https://www.cdc.gov/chronicdisease/resources/infographic/chronic-diseases.htm.

"take on the T-reg identity": Matt Richtel, *An Elegant Defense: The Extraordinary New Science of the Immune System: A Tale in Four Lives* (New York: William Morrow, 2019), 258.

That's because stress hormones signal: Richtel, *An Elegant Defense*, 266.

I'd simply expended all my chronic illness "spoons": "Spoon theory" is a metaphor for chronic illness written by Christine Miserandino about her life with lupus. People managing illness begin every day with a small reserve of energy: a certain number of spoonfuls available to expend. Often even small tasks draw upon our spoons, and we must ration them carefully from day to day—because once they're gone, they're gone. See "But You Don't Look Sick? Support for Those with Invisible Illness or Chronic Illness—The Spoon Theory," www.butyoudontlooksick.com/articles/written-by-christine/the-spoon-theory/, accessed February 1, 2022.

From my body to ancient writings: My language for God tends toward expanding, rather than limiting, our imaginations about God (but sometimes more traditional language better serves our purposes too). On occasion I refer to "Holy Spirit" as a name of one—the historically neglected one—of the three persons of the triune God. At times "the Holy Spirit" is more useful or, frankly, less distracting.

in the family of things: Mary Oliver, "Wild Geese," *Dream Work* (New York: Grove Atlantic, 2014), 11.

"sin is anything that breaks": Lisa Sharon Harper, *The Very Good Gospel: How Everything Wrong Can Be Made Right* (New York: Waterbrook, 2016), 48.

"God's dream for the world": Harper, *The Very Good Gospel*, 13.

When we speak of systemic change: adrienne maree brown, *Emergent Strategy: Shaping Changes, Changing Worlds* (Chico, CA: AK Press, 2017), 59–60.

CHAPTER 1: MY BODY AND OTHER CRUMBLING EMPIRES

"PHENOMENAL COSMIC POWER . . .": *Aladdin,* directed by Ron Clements and John Musker (1995; Buena Vista Pictures).

"I'd rather not see these people": Maya Dusenbery, *Doing Harm: The Truth About How Bad Medicine and Lazy Science Leave Women Dismissed, Misdiagnosed, and Sick,* e-reader ed. (New York: Harper-One, 2018), 367.

When another person made me angry: Annie Murphy Paul, *The Extended Mind: The Power of Thinking Outside the Brain* (Boston: Houghton Mifflin Harcourt, 2021), loc. 570.

CHAPTER 2: WHY WE NEED TO HEAL

It was hard to trust: I've chosen here to follow the lead of authors and scholars I respect, such as Osheta Moore, Dr. Chanequa Walker-Barnes, and Dr. Nell Painter in capitalizing the "W" in White. As Moore explains: "I ascribe to the idea that capitalizing Black but not White is another form of normalizing Whiteness. When White is the standard, then there's really no need to denote it. White is not the standard. Human is the standard." Osheta Moore, *Dear White Peacemakers: Dismantling Racism with Grit and Grace* (Harrisonburg, VA: Herald Press, 2021), 44–45. I'd add that when I feel uncomfortable with the capitalization, it is also because it seems to run the risk of creating a false equivalence between Black identities and cultures formed in the process of surviving the African diaspora and White identities and cultures created to consolidate privilege, power, and dominance. However, if the capitalization even simply invites us to think about these complexities, it's doing important work.

perhaps even barely human: Their mocking nickname for some neighboring people groups morphed into our English word "barbarian."

"In a profoundly sick society": Glennon Doyle, cited in Beverly Ford, "Glennon Doyle Shares How She Became a 'Warrior,'" July 19, 2019, https://coverage.bluecrossma.com/article/hubweek
-stories-glennon-doyle-shares-how-she-became-warrior.

Jesus says our greatest power: Here the usage of "empire" follows a short-hand some theologians use to talk about all forces of violence, oppression, and domination that have their roots in the logics, cultures, patterns, and systems of empires.

CHAPTER 3: AMERICAN HEALTHCARE AND OTHER OXYMORONS

I would later learn: Richtel, *An Elegant Defense*, 354.

CHAPTER 4: HEALING COMES FROM INSIDE OUT

Even though there is little: Space prohibits me from including more research about anti-fat bias; besides, as a straight-size person, there's only so much you can learn from me. The *Huffington Post* article "Everything You Know About Obesity Is Wrong" offers a great starting point grounded in empirical research, https://highline.huffingtonpost.com/articles/en/everything -you-know-about-obesity-is-wrong/. More resources are listed in the resources section.

Your intuition and your providers': Richtel, *The Extended Mind.*

"the next right thing": Emily P. Freeman, *The Next Right Thing: A Simple, Soulful Practice for Making Life Decisions* (Grand Rapids: Revell, 2019).

"it doesn't have to be this way": Andre Henry, "It Doesn't Have to Be This Way," from the album *Future Reggae* (2018).

CHAPTER 5: THE ECONOMY AND OTHER CONVENIENT FICTIONS

Chemically, we are unable: Emily Nagoski and Amelia Nagoski, *Burnout: The Secret to Unlocking the Stress Cycle* (New York: Ballantine Books, 2019), 5.

Beneath my many layers: In the disability community, many people use the phrase "sick and/or disabled" to denote that the experiences of illness and of disability are distinct in many ways, even though both groups of people contend with structural ableism in their day-to-day lives. Notably, people with mobility issues or neurodiverse brains, among others, are not in need of "healing" in the same way as many chronically ill people experience our own bodies to be.

As the disability community is inherently made up of people with widely diverse experiences, I tend to use the terms interchangeably for myself. In current usage, "disabled" more clearly expresses that I identify with a broad community of people who experience ableism, not just that I experience my own body as having illness.

"ordinary lives incorporate": Nancy L. Eiesland, *The Disabled God: Toward a Liberatory Theology of Disability*, 1st ed. (Nashville: Abingdon Press, 1994), 48.

"Our struggle against": Eiesland, *The Disabled God,* 86.

Eiesland calls this Jesus a **survivor:** Eiesland, *The Disabled God,* 102.

Jesus shows us that: Eiesland, *The Disabled God,* 103.

"is not an apology": Sonya Renee Taylor, *The Body Is Not an Apology: The Power of Radical Self-Love,* 2nd ed. (Oakland, CA: Berrett-Koehler Publishers, 2021).

"The disabled God embodies the ability": Eiesland, *The Disabled God,* 102.

CHAPTER 6: HEALING IS PRICELESS

The principle of essentialism: Greg McKeown, *Essentialism: The Disciplined Pursuit of Less* (New York: Crown, 2014).

CHAPTER 7: COMMUNITY AND OTHER RESCUED BUZZWORDS

The visceral sense of threat: Vivek H. Murthy, *Together: The Healing Power of Human Connection in a Sometimes Lonely World* (New York: Harper-Collins, 2020), loc. 812.

On the other hand: Nagoski and Nagoski, *Burnout,* 134.

"The 'common wisdom'": Nagoski and Nagoski, *Burnout,* 134–35.

Failing to be mirrored: Aundi Kolber, *Try Softer: A Fresh Approach to Move Us out of Anxiety, Stress, and Survival Mode—and into a Life of Connection and Joy* (Carol Stream, IL: Tyndale, 2020), 233, n. 2 of chap. 2.

CHAPTER 8: HEALING IS SHARED

Every role in the wide ecosystem: My emphasis in this chapter on "moving at the speed of trust," as adrienne maree brown says, to form community is influenced by a workshop with Kennae Miller of Charleston's Transformation Yoga called "In Agreement." The phrasing of "stepping forward and stepping back" is also borrowed from In Agreement.

After all, we are all only: David Radcliff, cited on Alie Ward's podcast *Ologies,* episode "Systems Biology with Emily E. Ackerman," August 3, 2021, https://www.alieward.com/ologies /systemsbiology.

CHAPTER 9: EARTH AND OTHER PRICELESS TRASH HEAPS

I was knee-deep: Robert D. Abbott, Adam Sadowski, and Angela G. Alt, "Efficacy of the Autoimmune Protocol Diet as Part of a Multi-Disciplinary, Supported Lifestyle Intervention for Hashimoto's Thyroiditis," *Cureus* 11, no. 4 (April 27, 2019), https://doi.org/10.7759/cureus.4556; Gauree G. Konijeti, et al.,

"Efficacy of the Autoimmune Protocol Diet for Inflammatory Bowel Disease," *Inflammatory Bowel Diseases* 23, no. 11 (November 2017): 2054–60, https://doi.org/10.1097/MIB.0000000000001221.

They could also be affected: Alexander Capuco, et al., "Current Perspectives on Gut Microbiome Dysbiosis and Depression," *Advances in Therapy 37*, no. 4 (April 2020): 1328–46, https://doi.org/10.1007/s12325-020-01272-7.

Spending time in green spaces: Paul, *The Extended Mind*, loc. 1726.

CHAPTER 10: FROM DISCONNECTION TO WHOLENESS

"Our movements themselves": Leah Lakshmi Piepzna-Samarasinha, "A Not-So-Brief Personal History of the Healing Justice Movement, 2010–2016," https://micemagazine.ca/issue-two /not-so-brief-personal-history-healing-justice-movement -2010%E2%80%932016.

I've made lots of friends: See Resources in the back of this book. "What we pay attention to grows": adrienne marie brown, "attention liberation," January 1, 2018, http://adriennemareebrown .net/2018/01/01/attention-liberation-a-commitment-a-year -of-practice/.

"the energy of all relationship": Rita Nakashima Brock, *Journeys by Heart: A Christology of Erotic Power* (New York: Crossroad, 1988), 41. Audre Lorde's "The Uses of the Erotic" became a foundational text for the concept of "the erotic" upon which Brock is drawing. Brock follows Huanani-Kay Trask and Susan Griffin in expanding somewhat upon Lorde's definition.

We have each been entrusted: I first heard this phrase years ago in a podcast interview with author Elizabeth Gilbert.

She speaks of Eros: Brock, *Journeys by Heart*, 109.

we need our work: brown, *Emergent Strategy*, 45.